A POCKET GUIDE
TO BASIC NURSING

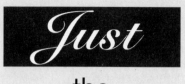

Just
the
Facts

A POCKET GUIDE
TO BASIC NURSING

Veronica Peterson
BA, RN, BSN, MS

University of Wisconsin Hospital and Clinics
Madison, Wisconsin

with 74 illustrations

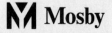 **Mosby**

St. Louis Baltimore Berlin Boston Carlsbad Chicago
London Madrid Naples New York Philadelphia
Sydney Tokyo Toronto

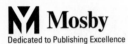
Mosby
Dedicated to Publishing Excellence

Editor: Susan Epstein
Developmental Editor: Beverly Copland
Project Manager: Karen Edwards
Production Editor: Stavra Demetrulias
Designer: Elizabeth Fett
Manufacturing Supervisor: Karen Lewis

Copyright © 1995 by Mosby–Year Book, Inc.

Printed in the United States of America
Composition by Clarinda Company
Printing/binding by R.R. Donnelley & Sons Company

Mosby–Year Book, Inc.
11830 Westline Industrial Drive
St. Louis, Missouri 63146

Library of Congress Cataloging in Publication Data

Peterson, Veronica.
    Just the facts : a pocket guide to basic nursing /
Veronica Peterson.
        p.   cm.
    Includes bibliographical references and index.
    ISBN 0-8016-7877-3
    1. Nursing—Handbooks, manuals, etc.   I. Title.
    [DNLM: 1. Nursing Care—handbooks.   WY 39 P485j
    1995]
RT51.P385   1995
610.73—dc20
DNLM/DLC
for Library of Congress   94-15043
                                                                      CIP

95 96 97 / 9 8 7 6 5 4 3 2

PREFACE

When I began my first student clinical experience I felt overwhelmed. There just wasn't time to memorize lab values, metric conversions, or the dozens of other facts I needed to know. So I compiled a small notebook of this information and carried it with me everywhere. Later, as a graduate student pursuing my master's degree, I taught nursing students who were experiencing the same problem.

For them, and for you, I have compiled those hard-to-memorize charts, graphs, numbers, and abbreviations that you must know, even in your first clinical experience. I've added some handy checklists for physical assessment and an assortment of other useful bits of information.

Just the Facts: a Pocket Guide to Basic Nursing is designed to be a portable, quick reference for facts and figures, focusing on adult health care. I hope you will find this as handy a resource during your clinical work as I did.

I would like to express my gratitude to the following people who reviewed this manuscript and offered suggestions and ideas: Lisa Bauer, RN, MS; Sue Hughes, RN, MS; Paula Jarzemsky, RN, MS; Patricia Emery Berry, RN, MS; Diana Girdley, RN, MSN; Patricia L. Roder, RN, MS; Kris Sippel, RN,

BSN; Rita R. Vosters, RN, MS; and Ann Windsor, RN, DNS, without whose encouragement this project might not have been completed.

Finally, I wish to thank my husband, Matthew, for his love, support, and most of all his encouragement.

Ronnie Peterson

CONTENTS

CHAPTER 1

Health Care Terminology

Abbreviations
Prefixes
Suffixes
Symbols
Medical Specialists
Nursing Specialties
Body Regions
Directions and Planes

For a more in-depth study of health care terminology consult the following publications:

Anderson KN, Anderson LE: *Mosby's pocket dictionary of medicine, nursing, and allied health,* St Louis, 1994, Mosby.
Austrin MG, Austrin HR: *Learning medical terminology,* ed 7, St Louis, 1991, Mosby.

ABBREVIATIONS*

ā before
aa of each
AAA abdominal aortic aneurysm
abd abdomen
ABG arterial blood gas
ac before meals
ACTH adrenocorticotropic hormone
ADH antidiuretic hormone
ADL activities of daily living
ad lib as desired
AIDS acquired immunodeficiency syndrome
AK above the knee
AKA above the knee amputation
ALS amyotrophic lateral sclerosis
am morning
ama against medical advice
amb ambulatory
amt amount
ANS autonomic nervous system
A&O alert and oriented
AODA alcohol and other drug abuse
A&P auscultation and percussion
Aq water
ARC AIDS-related complex
ARDS adult respiratory distress syndrome
ASA aspirin
AV atrioventricular
A&W alive and well

Ba barium
BBT basal body temperature
BE barium enema
bid twice per day
BK below the knee

*Standard abbreviations may vary by institution.

BKA below the knee amputation
BM bowel movement
BMR basal metabolic rate
BP blood pressure
BPH benign prostatic hypertrophy
BR bedrest
BRBPR bright red blood per rectum
BRP bathroom privileges
BS blood sugar; bowel sounds; breath sounds
BSA body surface area
BT bleeding time
BUN blood urea nitrogen
Bx biopsy

$\overline{\text{c}}$ with
C Celsius
C&A Clinitest and Acetest
Ca cancer
CABG coronary artery bypass graft
CAD coronary artery disease
CAT computerized axial tomography
CBC complete blood count
CBI continuous bladder irrigation
cbr complete bedrest
CBS chronic brain syndrome
CC chief complaint
cc cubic centimeter
CCU coronary care unit
CDC Centers for Disease Control and Prevention
cg centigram
CHD coronary heart disease
CHF congestive heart failure
CHO carbohydrate
Cl chlorine
cl clear liquid diet
cm centimeter

cm³ cubic centimeter
CMV cytomegalovirus
CNS central nervous system
c/o complains of
CO carbon monoxide
CO₂ carbon dioxide
COPD chronic obstructive pulmonary disease
CPK creatine phosphokinase
crit hematocrit
C&S culture and sensitivity
CS central supply; central service
c-sec cesarean section
CSF cerebrospinal fluid
CST convulsive shock therapy
CT computerized tomography
CVA cerebral vascular accident
CVP central venous pressure
CVS cardiovascular system
CXR chest x-ray
cysto cystoscopy

d day
DAT diet as tolerated
D&C dilatation and curettage
D/C discharge
dc discontinue
DDS doctor of dental surgery
DIC disseminated intravascular coagulation
diff differential blood count
DJD degenerative joint disease
DM diabetes mellitus
DNR do not resuscitate
DOA dead on arrival
DOB date of birth
DOE dyspneic on exertion
DTP diphtheria, tetanus, pertussis (vaccine)

DTR deep tendon reflex
DVT deep vein thrombosis
D₅W 5% dextrose in water
dx diagnosis

EBL estimated blood loss
EBV Epstein-Barr virus
ECF extracellular fluid
ECG electrocardiogram
ECT electroconvulsive therapy
ED effective dose
EDD estimated date of delivery
EEG electroencephalogram
(E)ENT (eye) ear, nose, throat
EKG electrocardiogram
EMG electromyogram
eom extraocular movement
esp extrasensory perception
ESRD end-stage renal disease
EST electroshock therapy
ETOH ethyl alcohol

F Fahrenheit
FBS fasting blood sugar
f/c/s fever, chills, sweats
FEV forced expiratory volume
FF force fluids
FHR fetal heart rate
Fl fluid; full liquid diet
FOB foot of the bed
FSH follicle-stimulating hormone
FUO fever of unknown origin
fx family; fracture
fx hx family history

g gram
GB gallbladder

GC gonococcus
GI gastrointestinal
gm gram
GP general practitioner
gr grain
grav I, II, III pregnancy one, two, three, etc.
GT gastrostomy tube
GTH gonadotropic hormone
gtt drops
GTT glucose tolerance test
GU genitourinary
GYN gynecology

h hour
HA headache
HAV hepatitis A virus
Hb hemoglobin
HBV hepatitis B virus
HCG human chorionic gonadotropin
Hct hematocrit
HGH human growth hormone
H&H hemoglobin and hematocrit
HIV human immunodeficiency virus (AIDS)
HLA human leukocyte antigen
HO house officer
HOB head of the bed
hr hour
hs at bedtime
HSV herpes simplex virus
HTN hypertension
HVD hypertensive vascular disease
hypo hypodermic
hx history

IC inspiratory capacity
ICP intracranial pressure
ICS intercostal space

ICU intensive care unit
I&D incision and drainage
IDDM insulin-dependent diabetes mellitus
IE immunoelectrophoresis
Ig immunoglobulin
IH infectious hepatitis
IM intramuscular
I&O intake and output
IOP intraocular pressure
IP intraperitoneal
IPPB intermittent positive pressure breathing (device)
Irr irregular
IUD intrauterine device
IV intravenous
IVP intravenous push
IVPB intravenous piggyback

JRA juvenile rheumatoid arthritis
JVD jugular vein distention
JVP jugular vein pressure

K+ potassium
kg kilogram
KUB kidney, ureter, bladder
KVO keep vein open

L left; liter
lat lateral
LBBB left bundle branch block
LCM left costal margin
LD lethal dose
LE lower extremity
LFT liver function tests
LGH lactogenic hormone
LH luteinizing hormone
LLL left lower lobe

LLQ left lower quadrant
LMP last menstrual period
LOC level of consciousness; loss of consciousness
LP lumbar puncture
LPN licensed practical nurse
LS lumbosacral
LSB left sternal border
LUL left upper lobe
LUQ left upper quadrant
LVH left ventricular hypertrophy

m meter
M murmur
MAP mean arterial pressure
MD medical doctor
MED minimal effective dose
mEq milliequivalent
Mg magnesium
mg milligram
MG myasthenia gravis
MI myocardial infarction
ml milliliter
mm millimeter
MM mucous membrane
mm^3 cubic millimeter
mm Hg millimeters of mercury
MRI magnetic resonance imaging
MS multiple sclerosis
MSL midsternal line
MSO$_4$ morphine sulfate

Na sodium
NAD no appreciable disease
NAS no added salt
NIDDM noninsulin-dependent diabetes mellitus
NIH National Institutes of Health
ng nasogastric

NKDA no known drug allergies
noc night
NPN nonprotein nitrogen
NPO nothing by mouth
NS normal saline
N&V nausea and vomiting

OB obstetrics
OBS organic brain syndrome
OD overdose; right eye
OM otitis media
OOB out of bed
OR operating room
ORIF open reduction (with) internal fixation
OS left eye
OT occupational therapy
OTC over the counter
OU both eyes

p after
PA physician's assistant
P&A posterior and anterior
Paco$_2$ partial pressure of carbon dioxide (arterial)
Pao$_2$ partial pressure of oxygen (arterial)
Pap Papanicolaou test
PAR postanesthesia room
pat paroxysmal atrial tachycardia
pc after meals
PCA patient-controlled analgesia
PCN penicillin
Pco$_2$ partial pressure of carbon dioxide
PCV packed cell volume
PCWP pulmonary capillary wedge pressure
PD postural drainage
PDR Physician's Desk Reference
PE physical exam; pulmonary emboli

PEEP positive end expiratory pressure
PEG pneumoencephalogram
PERRLA pupils equal, round, reactive to light, and accommodating
PET positron emission tomography
pH hydrogen ion concentration
PID pelvic inflammatory disease
PIH pregnancy-induced hypertension
PKU phenylketonuria
pm afternoon
PM post mortem
PMH past medical history
PMS premenstrual syndrome
po by mouth
Po$_2$ partial pressure of oxygen
poly many
pr per rectum
prn as needed
pt patient
PT physical therapy
PTT partial thromboplastin time
PUD peptic ulcer disease
PVC premature ventricular contraction

q every
qd every day
qh every hour
q2h, q3h, etc. every 2 hours, every 3 hours, etc.
qhs every evening
qid four times a day
ql as much as desired
qn every night
qns quantity not sufficient
qod every other day
qs quantity sufficient

R right
RA rheumatoid arthritis
rad radiation absorbed dose
RBBB right bundle branch block
RBC red blood cells; red blood count
RCM right costal margin
RDA recommended daily allowance
REM rapid eye movement
rep repeat
RF rheumatic fever
Rh rhesus factor
RHD rheumatic heart disease
RLL right lower lobe
RLQ right lower quadrant
RML right middle lobe
RN registered nurse
R/O rule out
ROM range of motion
ROS review of systems
RR respiratory rate
RRR regular rate and rhythm
RT respiratory therapy
RUL right upper lobe
RUQ right upper quadrant
RVH right ventricular hypertrophy
Rx treatment

s without
SB sternal border
SBO small bowel obstruction
SC subcutaneous
SD skin dose
SIDS sudden infant death syndrome
sig let it be labeled
SL under the tongue
SLE systemic lupus erythematosus

SOB short of breath
SOS if necessary
S/P status post
sp gr specific gravity
SQ subcutaneous
sr sedimentation rate
ss a half
ST let it stand
STAT immediately
STD sexually transmitted disease
STS serologic for syphilis
SVT supraventricular tachycardia
sx symptom

T$_3$ triiodothyronine
T$_4$ tetraiodothyronine (thyroxine)
T&A tonsillectomy and adenoidectomy
TAH total abdominal hysterectomy
TB tuberculosis
TBG thyroxin-binding globulin
TBI total body irradiation
tbsp tablespoon
T&C type and crossmatch
TCDB turn, cough, deep breathe
tea teaspoon
TG triglyceride
TIA transient ischemic attack
TIBC total iron-binding capacity
tid three times a day
TKO to keep open
TLC total lung capacity
TM tympanic membrane
TPN total parenteral nutrition
TPR temperature, pulse, respiration
TSA tumor-specific antigen
TSH thyroid-stimulating hormone

tsp teaspoon
TST triple sugar iron test
TURP transurethral resection of the prostate
tus cough
twe tap water enema

U unit
UA urinalysis
UA/UC urinalysis with culture
URI upper respiratory infection
US ultrasound
USP United States Pharmacopeia
ut dict as directed
UTI urinary tract infection

VA visual acuity
VC vital capacity
VD venereal disease
VDH valvular disease (of the) heart
VDRL Venereal Disease Research Laboratory (test for syphilis)
VF field of vision
VO verbal order
VR vocal resonance
VS vital signs
VSD ventricular septal defect
VT tidal volume
VW vessel wall

w watt
WBC white blood cells; white blood count
w/c wheelchair
WD well developed
WN well nourished
WNL within normal limits
WR Wassermann reactions
W/V weight in volume

PREFIXES

a, an absent
ab away from
ad to, toward
aer air
ambi, ampho both
ana up, toward
angi(o) blood vessel
ante before
ap, apo separation
arteri(o) artery
aud ear
aut, aut(o) self

bi two
brady slow

cardi(o) heart
cata down, under
cephal(o) head
cerebr(o) brain
chole gallbladder
chondr(o) cartilage
circum around
cirrh(o) yellow
co, con with, together
colo colon
contra opposed
cost(o) rib
cran head
crani(o) skull
cyan(o) blue
cyst(o) liquid filled, urinary, bladder

dactyl(o) fingers, toes
de down, from

dent(o) teeth
derma skin
di two, twice
dia between, apart
dis away, separate
dys bad, difficult

e, ec, ex away from
ect, ecto outer, outside
em, en in
endo within, inside
enter(o) intestines
epi on, over
erythr(o) red
eu normal, well
extra outside of

gastr(o) stomach
glyc(o) sugar

hem, hemato blood
hemi half
hepat(o) liver
hyper above, beyond
hypo beneath, below

ile(o) ileum
ili(o) ilium
im, in in, into
infra below
inter between
intra within

leuk(o) white
lingu(o) tongue
lip(o) fat
lith(o) stone

macro large
mal bad
mega large
melan(o) black
micro small
mono one
multi many
my(o) muscle
myel(o) bone marrow, spinal cord

nephr(o) kidney
neur(o) nervous system

ophthalm(o) eye
oste(o) bone
ot(o) ear

pan all, entire
para, par beside, near
per through
peri around
phag(o) eat
phleb(o) vein
pneum(o) lung
poli(o) gray matter
poly many

post after
pre before
proct(o) rectal
pseudo false
psych(o) the mind

re back, again
ren(o) kidney
retro backward
rhin(o) nose

semi half
splen(o) spleen
spondyl(o) spinal cord
sub below
super, supra above
sym, syn together

tachy fast
tetra four
trans across
tri three

uni one
ultra beyond

vas(o) blood vessel
ven(o) vein

SUFFIXES

ac, al pertaining to
algia pain
ate, ize use, subject to

cele protrusion
centesis puncture to remove fluid
cle, cule small
cyte cell

dynia pain

ectomy removal
emia blood condition
ent, er, ist person
esis, tion condition

form, oid resembling

genic, genesis origin
gram, graph written record

ia, ism, ity condition
iasis presence of
ible, ile capable
ites, itis inflammation

logy study of

megaly enlargement

ola, ole small
oma tumor
osis, sis abnormal condition

ostomy opening
ous, tic pertaining to
oxia oxygen

pathy disease
penia deficiency of
pexy, pexis fixation
phagia, phagy eating
phobia fear
plasty surgical shaping
pnea breathing
ptosis prolapse downward

rrhage, rrhagia excessive flow
rrhaphy suturing in place
rrhea flow, discharge
rrhexis rupture

scope, tome examination instrument
scopy examination
stomy surgical opening

tony incision

ule, ulum, ulus small
uria urine

SYMBOLS

⚲ standing
ᑫ sitting
○– laying
↑ increasing
↓ decreasing
R right
L left
♀ female
♂ male
ʒ dram
℥ ounce
° degree
′ minute
°C Celsius
°F Fahrenheit
♏ minim

× times
= equal to
< less than
≤ less than or equal to
> greater than
≥ greater than or equal to
≈ about
Ø none or no
→ leading to
@ at
ṫ ṫṫ ṫṫṫ one, two, three
number
″ seconds
μg microgram
μm micrometer

MEDICAL SPECIALISTS

Allergist treats the body's reactions to unusual sensitivity

Anesthesiologist treats with anesthesia

Cardiologist treats conditions and diseases of the heart and blood vessels

Dermatologist treats conditions and diseases of the skin

Endocrinologist treats conditions and diseases of the endocrine system

Family practitioner treats clients of all ages with medical methods

Gastroenterologist treats conditions and diseases of the digestive tract

General practitioner treats clients of all ages with medical methods

Geneticist specialist in the study of genetics

Gerontologist treats conditions and diseases related to the elderly

Gynecologist treats conditions and diseases of the female reproductive system

Hematologist treats blood disorders

Internist treats nonsurgical conditions and diseases in adults and children

Neonatologist treats conditions and diseases in newborns

Neurologist treats conditions and diseases of the brain, spinal cord, and nerves

Neurosurgeon treats conditions and diseases of the brain, spinal cord, and nerves with surgical methods

Obstetrician treats women during pregnancy and postpartum

Oncologist treats tumors (cancers) with surgical and medical methods

Ophthalmologist treats conditions and diseases of the eye

Orthopedist treats conditions and diseases of the muscles and bones

Otolaryngologist treats conditions and diseases of the ears, nose, and throat

Pathologist diagnoses conditions and diseases through changes in tissues

Pediatrician treats conditions and diseases in children

Plastic surgeon treats or restores structural conditions by corrective surgery

Podiatrist treats conditions and diseases of the foot

Psychiatrist treats mental disorders

Radiologist treats conditions and diseases with radiant energy

Rheumatologist treats conditions and diseases of the muscles and joints

Surgeon treats conditions and diseases with surgical methods

Thoracic surgeon surgically treats conditions and diseases of the chest cavity

Urologist treats conditions and diseases of the kidneys, bladder, ureters, and male reproductive system

NURSING SPECIALTIES

ADN associate degree nurse

BS (BSN) bachelor of science or bachelor of science in nursing

CCRN critical care registered nurse

CEN certified emergency nurse

CNM clinical nurse manager

CNS clinical nurse specialist

CRNA certified registered nurse anesthetist

DSN doctor of science in nursing

EdD doctorate of education

LPN licensed practical nurse

LVN licensed vocational nurse

MEd master of education

MPH master of public health

MS (MSN) master of science or master of science in nursing

MSNR master of science in nursing with research

NP nurse practitioner

OCN oncology certified nurse

ONS oncology nurse specialist

PhD (PhDc) doctor of philosophy or doctoral candidate

RNC registered nurse certified

TNCC trauma nurse core course (certification)

BODY REGIONS

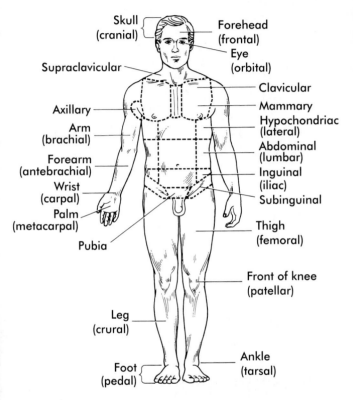

Figure 1-1 Anterior body regions.

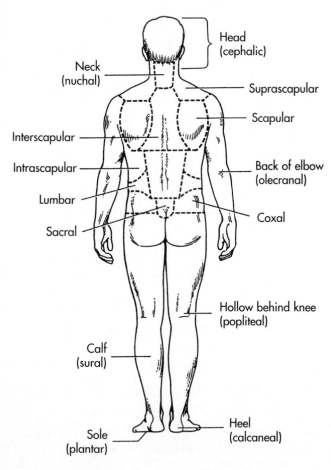

Figure 1-2   Posterior body regions.

DIRECTIONS AND PLANES

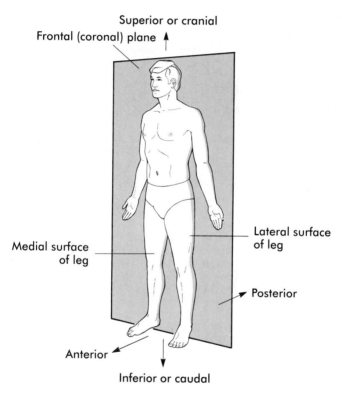

Figure 1-3 Frontal and lateral planes. (From Austrin MG, Austrin HR: *Learning medical terminology,* ed 7, St Louis, 1991, Mosby.)

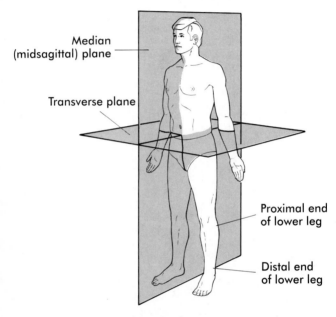

Figure 1-4 Medial and transverse planes. (From Austrin MG, Austrin HR: *Learning medical terminology,* ed 7, St Louis, 1991, Mosby.)

CHAPTER 2

Medications: Calculations and Administration

For a more in-depth study of medications: calculations and administration consult the following publications:

Gray DC: *Calculate with confidence*, St Louis, 1994, Mosby.
Potter PA, Perry AG: *Fundamentals of nursing: concepts, process, and practice*, ed 3, St Louis, 1993, Mosby.
Skidmore-Roth L: *Mosby's 1994 nursing drug reference*, St Louis, 1994, Mosby.

EQUIVALENT MEASURES

Metric System

Rules

To change from a larger to smaller unit MULTIPLY the number by 10, 100, etc or move the decimal to the RIGHT. To change from a smaller to larger unit DIVIDE the number by 10, 100, etc. or move the decimal to the LEFT.

Weight

1 kilogram (kg/Kg) = 1000 grams (gm)
1 gram (Gm/gm/g/G) = 1000 milligrams (mg)
1 milligram (mg) = 1000 micrograms (mcg)

Volume

1 liter (L) = 1000 milliliters (ml)
1 deciliter (dl) = 100 milliliters (ml)
1 milliliter (ml) = 1 cubic centimeter (cc)

Length

1 meter (m) = 100 centimeters (cm)
1 meter (m) = 1000 millimeters (mm)
1 centimeter (cm) = 10 millimeters (mm)

Apothecary System

Weight: grains (gr); Volume: minims (m); drams (dr); ounces (oz)

Rules

Metric to Apothecary Conversions:
Grams to grains: multiply grams (gm) by 15
Milligrams to grains: divide milligrams (mg) by 60

Apothecary to Metric Conversions:
Grains to grams: divide grains (gr) by 15
Grains to milligrams: multiply grains (gr) by 60

Household System

Weight

1 tablespoon (Tbsp/T) = 3 teaspoons (tsp/t)
1 cup (c) = 16 tablespoons (Tbsp/T)
1 pound (lb) = 16 ounces (oz)

Volume

1 gallon (gal) = 4 quarts (qt)
1 quart (qt) = 2 pints (pt)
1 pint (pt) = 2 cups (c)
1 cup (c) = 8 ounces (oz)

Kilogram to Pound Conversions:
Kilograms to pounds: multiply kilograms (kg) by 2.2
Pounds to kilograms: divide pounds (lb) by 2.2

PEDIATRIC BODY SURFACE AREA

$$\text{Child's dose} = \frac{\text{Child's BSA in square meters} \times \text{adult dose}}{1.7}$$

CALCULATING STRENGTH OF A SOLUTION

Solution Strength: Desired Solution:

$$\frac{X}{100} = \frac{\text{Amount of drug desired}}{\text{Amount of finished solution}}$$

CALCULATING IV DRIP RATES

The drops per 1 ml is the number of drops needed to fill a 1 ml syringe

The rate is the number of ml per hour

The drip rate is the amount of volume divided by the time needed to infuse

Below is the equation that can be used to calculate IV drip rates:

$$\frac{\text{Total volume}}{\text{Total time}} = \frac{\text{ml}}{1 \text{ minute}} \times \frac{\text{number of gtt}}{\text{ml}} = \frac{\text{drops}}{\text{minute}}$$

Microdrops: a Simple Calculation

10 drops or gtt: ml/hr = gtt/min per micro divided by 6

15 drops or gtt: ml/hr = gtt/min per micro divided by 4

20 drops or gtt: ml/hr = gtt/min per micro divided by 3

60 drops or gtt/ml: ml/hr = gtt/min

DRUG ADMINISTRATION

Routes of Administration

Oral (PO), sublingual (SL), rectal (PR), topical (T), subcutaneous (SQ), intramuscular (IM), intravenous (IV), inhalation (IH).

Six Rights

Client, drug, dose, time, route, documentation.

Types of Drug Preparations

Aerosol spray; capsule (coated); cream (nongreasy); elixir (alcohol); extract (concentrated); gel (clear, semisolid); liniment (oily); lotion; lozenge; ointment (semisolid); paste (thicker than ointment); pills powder (ground drug); spirit (alcohol); suppository (dissolves at body temperature); syrup (sugar-based); tablet (coated); tincture (alcohol).

Therapeutic Drugs

Palliative relieves symptoms; example: pain medications

Curative cures disease; example: antibiotics

Supportive helps body's functions; example: blood pressure medications

Destructive destroys cells; example: chemotherapy

Restorative returns body to health; example: vitamins

Common Allergic Responses

Difficulty breathing, palpitations, hives (urticaria), skin rashes (eczema), nausea, vomiting, pruritus, rhinitis, tearing, wheezing, diarrhea. *Report all allergic responses.*

Common Drug Terminology

Biotransformation chemical alteration of a compound from one form to another

Distribution where drug is taken up into the body tissues

Duration length of time drug remains in the body

Half-life time required for one half of the remaining drug to be eliminated from the body

Idiosyncratic property of drug that cannot be predicted

Onset first response of drug in the body

Peak highest level of drug in the body

Pharmacokinetics study of how drugs enter the body, reach their site of action, are metabolized, and exit the body

Plateau concentration of scheduled doses

Side effects unintended secondary effects of drug

Therapeutic beneficial effect and level of drug

Tolerance need for increased amount of drug to produce the same effect

Toxic nonbeneficial or lethal level of drug

Trough lowest level of drug in the body

THERAPEUTIC DRUGS THAT REQUIRE SERUM DRUG LEVELS*

Antibiotics
amikacin (Amikin)
gentamicin (Garamycin)
netilmicin (Netromycin)
tobramycin (Nebcin)
vancomycin (Vancocin)

Anticonvulsants
carbamazepine (Tegretol)
phenobarbital
phenytoin (Dilantin)
primidone (Mysoline)
valproic acid

Cardiovascular Drugs
digoxin (Lanoxin)
lidocaine (Xylocaine)
procainamide (Pronestyl)
quinidine

Respiratory Drug
theophylline

Antirejection Drug
cyclosporine

*Specific therapeutic blood levels may vary per facility.

Drug Compatibility Chart

	Atropine	Butorphanol	Chlordiazepoxide	Chlorpromazine	Codeine	Diazepam	Dimenhydrinate	Diphenhydramine	Droperidol	Fentanyl	Glycopyrrolate
Atropine		C	I	C		I	C	C	C	C	C
Butorphanol	C		I	C		I	I	C	C	C	
Chlordiazepoxide	I	I		I	I	I	I	I	I	I	I
Chlorpromazine	C	C	I			I	I	C	C	C	C
Codeine			I			I					
Diazepam	I	I	I	I	I		I	I	I	I	I
Dimenhydrinate	C	I	I	I		I		C	C	C	I
Diphenhydramine	C	C	I	C		I	C		C	C	C
Droperidol	C	C	I	C		I	C	C		C	C
Fentanyl	C	C	I	C		I	C	C	C		C
Glycopyrrolate	C		I	C		I	I	C	C	C	
Hydroxyzine	C	C	I	C		I	I	C	C	C	C
Innovar	C	C	I	C		I	C	C	C	C	C
Lorazepam	I	I	I	I	I	I	I	I	I	I	I
Meperidine	C	C	I	C		I	C	C	C	C	C
Metoclopramide	C	C	I	C		I	C	C	C	C	
Morphine	C	C	I	C		I	C	C	C	C	C
Nalbuphine	C		I			I			C		
Pentazocine	C	C	I	C		I	C	C	C	C	I
Pentobarbital	C	I	I	I	I	I	I	I	I	I	I
Perphenazine	C	C	I	C		I	C	C	C	C	
Prochlorperazine	C	C	I	C		I	I	C	C	C	C
Promazine	C		I	C		I	I	C	C	C	C
Promethazine	C	C	I	C		I	I	C	C	C	C
Scopolamine Hbr	C	C	I	G		I	C	C	C	C	C
Secobarbital	I	I	I	I	I	I	I	I	I	I	I
Thiethylperazine		C	I			I					
Trimethobenzamide			I			I					C

Developed by Providence Memorial Hospital, El Paso, Texas. From Skidmore-Roth L; *Mosby's nursing drug reference,* ed 6, St. Louis, 1993, Mosby. NOTE: Give within 15 minutes of mixing. C, compatible; I, incompatible; □, no documented information.

Hydroxyzine	Innovar	Lorazepam	Meperidine	Metoclopramide	Morphine	Nalbuphine	Pentazocine	Pentobarbital	Perphenazine	Prochlorperazine	Promazine	Promethazine	Scopolamine Hbr	Secobarbital	Thiethylperazine	Trimethobenzamide
C	C	I	C	C	C	C	C	C	C	C	C	C	C	I		
C	C	I	C	C	C		C	I	C	C		C	C	I	C	
I	I	I	I	I	I	I	I	I	I	I	I	I	I	I	I	I
C	C	I	C	C	C		C	I	C	C	C	C	C	I		
	I						I						I			
I	I	I	I	I	I	I	I	I	I	I	I	I	I	I	I	I
I	C	I	C	C	C		C	I	C	I	I	I	C	I		
C	C	I	C	C	C	C	C	I	C	C	C	C	C	I		
C	C	I	C	C	C	C	C	I	C	C	C	C	C	I		
C	C	I	C	C	C		C	I	C	C	C	C	C	I		
C	C	I	C		C		I	I		C	C	C	C	I		C
	C	I	C	C	C	C	C	I		C	C	C	C	I		
C		I	C	C	C	C	C	I	C	C	C	C	C	I		
I	I		I	I	I	I	I	I	I	I	I	I	I	I	I	I
C	C	I		C	I		C	I	C	C	C	C	C	I		
C	C	I	C		C		C		C	C	C	C	C	I		
C	C	I	I	C			C	I	C	C	C	C	C	I		
C	C	I					I		C		C	C	I	C	C	
C	C	I	C	C	C			I	C	C	C	C	C	I		
I	I	I	I		I	I	I		I	I	I	I	C	I		
	C	I	C	C	C		C	I		C		C	C	I	I	
C	C	I	C	C	C	C	C	I	C		C	C	C	I		
C	C	I	C	C	C		C	I		C		C	C	I		
C	C	I	C	C	C	C	C	I	C	C	C		C	I		
C	C	I	C	C	C	C	C	C	C	C	C	C		I		
I	I	I	I	I	I	I	I	I	I	I	I	I	I	I		I
		I			C			I						I		
		I			C									I		

Parenteral compatibility occurs when two or more drugs are successfully mixed without liquefaction, deliquescence, or precipitation.

ADMINISTRATION TECHNIQUES

Injection Guide for Needle Size and Volume		
		Volume Injected (ml)
Needle Sizes	**Average**	**Range**
Intradermal	26 or 27 gauge × ⅜ in	0.1	0.001-1.0
Subcutaneous	25-27 gauge × ½ to ⅝ in	0.5	0.5-1.5
Intramuscular			
Gluteus medius	20-23 gauge × 1½ to 3 in	2-4	1-5
Gluteus minimus	20-23 gauge × 1½ to 3 in	1-4	1-5
Vastus lateralis	22-25 gauge × ⅝ to 1 in	1-4	1-5
Deltoid	23-25 gauge × ⅝ to 1 in	0.5	0.5-2
Intravenous bolus	18-23 gauge × 1 to 1½ in	1-10	0.5-50 (or more by continuous infusion)

From Myers JL: *Quick medication administration reference*, St Louis, 1992, Mosby.

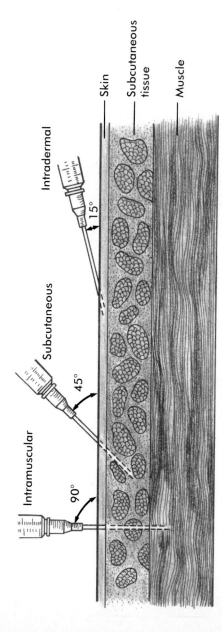

Figure 2-1 Angles of injections. (From Potter PA, Perry AG: *Fundamentals of nursing,* ed 3, St Louis, 1993, Mosby.)

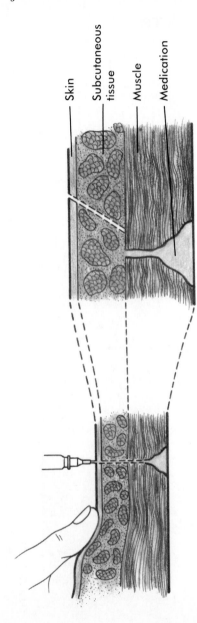

Figure 2-2 Z-track injection. (From Potter PA, Perry AG: *Fundamentals of nursing,* ed 3, St Louis, 1993, Mosby.)

INJECTION SITES

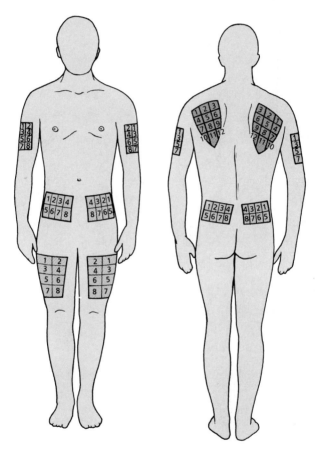

Figure 2-3 Common sites for subcutaneous injections. (From Potter PA, Perry AG: *Fundamentals of nursing*, ed 3, St Louis, 1993, Mosby.)

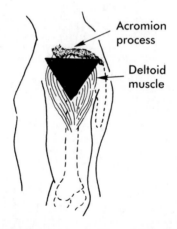

Figure 2-4   Deltoid injections. (From Myers JL: *Quick medication administration reference,* St Louis, 1992, Mosby.)

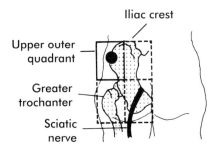

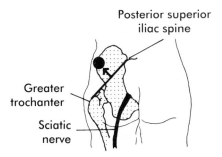

Figure 2-5   Dorsogluteal injections. (From Myers JL: *Quick medication administration reference,* St Louis, 1992, Mosby.)

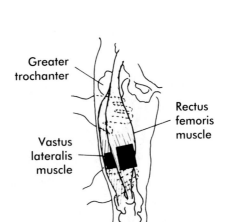

Figure 2-6   Vastus lateralis injections. (From Myers JL: *Quick medication administration reference,* St Louis, 1992, Mosby.)

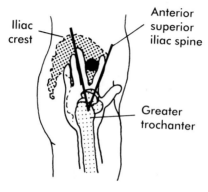

Figure 2-7 Ventrogluteal injections. (From Myers, JL: *Quick medication administration reference,* St Louis, 1992, Mosby.)

Infection Control

For a more in-depth study of infection control consult the following publications:

Anderson KN, Anderson LE: *Mosby's pocket dictionary of medicine, nursing, and allied health,* St Louis, 1994, Mosby.

Benenson AB, editor: *Control of communicable diseases in man,* Washington, D.C., 1990, American Public Health Association.

Potter PA, Perry AG: *Fundamentals of nursing: concepts, process, and practice,* ed 3, St Louis, 1993, Mosby.

Universal precautions for prevention of transmission of human immunodeficiency virus, hepatitis B virus, and other bloodborne pathogens in health care settings, *MMWR* 37(suppl 24):377, 1988.

BASIC TERMS

Asepsis prevention of the transfer of microorganisms and pathogens

Chain infection's path; the components of the infectious disease process

Clean presence of few microorganisms or pathogens with no visible debris

Colonization presence of a potentially infectious organism in or on a host but not causing disease

Communicable ability of a microorganism to spread disease

Contamination presence of an infectious agent on a surface

Dirty presence of many microorganisms or pathogens; any soiled item

Disease alteration of normal tissues, body processes, or function

Etiology cause of a disease

Immunity resistance to a disease associated with the presence of antibodies

Infection invasion of tissues by a disease-causing microorganism(s)

Medical asepsis measures that limit pathologic spread of microorganisms

Nosocomial infection a hospital-acquired infection (not present or incubating on admission)

Ports how microorganisms exit and enter a system

Reservoir storage place for organisms to grow

Source point that initiates chain of infection

Sterile absence of all microorganisms

Surgical asepsis measures to keep pathogenic organisms at a minimum during surgery

Transmission method by which microorganisms travel from one host to another

Virulence ability of a microorganism to produce disease

STAGES OF INFECTION

Incubation from initial contact with infectious material to onset of symptoms

Prodrome from nonspecific signs and symptoms to specific signs and symptoms

Illness presence of specific signs and symptoms

Convalescence during the recovery period, as symptoms subside

THE INFLAMMATORY PROCESS

Stage I

Constriction of blood vessels, dilatation of small vessels, increased vessel permeability; increased leukocytes; swelling and pain. Leukocytes begin to engulf the infection.

Stage II

Exudation with fluids and dead cells.

Serous clear; part of the blood

Purulent thick; pus with leukocytes

Sanguineous bloody

Stage III

Repair of tissues. Examples include:

Regeneration same tissues

Stroma connective tissues

Parenchyma functional part

Fibrous scar

UNIVERSAL PRECAUTIONS

All blood and body fluids are considered to be potentially infectious.

Body Fluids to Which Universal Precautions *Always* Apply

Blood, serum, plasma, spinal fluid, pleural fluid, amniotic fluid, synovial fluid, vitreous fluid, pericardial fluid, semen, peritoneal fluid, vaginal secretions, wound exudate, and saliva (in dental procedures).

Body Fluids to Which Universal Precautions Apply When Blood is Visible

Sweat, tears, sputum, saliva, nasal secretions, feces, urine, vomitus, and breast milk.

Summary of Universal Precaution Recommendations

Hand washing should be done before and after working with all clients and after removing gloves; immediately if hands become contaminated with blood or other body fluids

Gloves should be worn whenever contact with body fluids is likely

Mask and/or eye cover should be worn when splashing of body fluids is likely

Gown should be worn when soiling of exposed skin or clothing is likely

CPR should be done using pocket masks or mechanical ventilation, avoiding mouth to mouth

Needles should not be recapped unless using the one-handed method;

DON'T BREAK NEEDLES; DISCARD ALL SHARP OBJECTS IMMEDIATELY

Spills should be cleaned immediately with bleach and water (one part bleach to nine parts water) or FDA-approved cleaning agent

Specimens should be collected using leakproof, puncture-resistant container; outside of container must be free of contaminants

TYPES OF ISOLATION

Isolation practices vary according to hospital policy. The categories below are taken from the Centers for Disease Control and Prevention's guidelines for infection control. *All* persons in isolation still require Universal Precautions.

Blood and Body Fluid Isolation

Prevents transmission of disease by direct or indirect contact with blood or body fluids. Uses include AIDS and hepatitis B.

Needs. Private room (only if poor hygiene); gloves for handling body fluids.

Contact Isolation

Prevents transmission of disease by direct contact. Uses include respiratory infections and wound infections.

Needs. Private room; mask (if near client); gown and gloves if in direct contact with infected area.

Drainage/Secretion Isolation

Prevents transmission of disease by direct or indirect contact. Used for skin infections.

Needs. Gown and gloves if in direct contact with infected areas.

Enteric Isolation

Prevents transmission by contact with feces. Uses include hepatitis.

Needs. Private room if incontinent; gown if soiling of clothing is likely; gloves for contact with feces.

Immunocompromised Isolation

Protects those with lowered immunity. Uses include organ transplant recipients.

Needs. Private room; masks when in contact with the client

Respiratory Isolation

Prevents airborne transmission. Uses include measles, mumps, and meningitis.

Needs. Private room; mask if working close to infected client

Strict Isolation

Prevents airborne or direct transmission. Uses include diphtheria.

Needs. Private room, closed door, gloves, gown, and mask

Tuberculosis (AFB) Isolation

Prevents transmission of acid-fast bacilli.

Needs. Private room with special ventilation; mask; gown if soiling is likely; gloves if in direct contact with infected client

COMMON BACTERIA*

Ear *Corynebacterium,* diphtheroids, saprophytes, *Staphylococcus, Streptococcus*

Esophagus/stomach None; usually microorganisms from the mouth or food

Eye *Corynebacterium, Enterobacter, Haemophilus, Moraxella, Neisseria, Staphylococcus, Streptococcus*

Genitalia *Bacteroides, Candida albicans, Corynebacterium,* enterococcus, *Fusobacterium, Mycobacterium, Mycoplasma, Neisseria, Staphylococcus, Streptococcus*

Ileum (lower) *Bacteroides, Clostridium, Enterobacter,* enterococcus, *Lactobacillus, Mycobacterium, Staphylococcus*

Ileum (upper) enterococcus, *Lactobacillus*

Large intestine *Acinetobacter, Actinomyces, Alcaligenes, Bacteroides, Clostridium, Enterobacter,* enterococcus, *Eubacterium, Fusobacterium, Mycobacterium, Peptococcus, Peptostreptococcus*

Mouth *Actinomyces, Bacteroides, Candida albicans, Corynebacterium, Enterobacter, Fusobacterium, Lactobacillus, Peptococcus, Peptostreptococcus, Staphylococcus, Streptococcus, Torulopsis, Veillonella*

Nose *Corynebacterium, Enterobacter, Haemophilus, Moraxella, Neisseria, Staphylococcus, Streptococcus*

Oropharynx *Corynebacterium, Enterobacter, Haemophilus, Staphylococcus, Streptococcus*

Skin *Bacillus, Candida albicans, Corynebacterium,* dermatophytes, *Enterobacter, Peptococcus, Propionibacterium acnes, Staphylococcus, Streptococcus*

*Normal flora found on or in the body.

TUBERCULOSIS

Agent
Mycobacterium tuberculosis
Bovine TB *(Mycobacterium bovis)* transmitted
through cattle and unpasteurized milk

Reservoir
Primarily humans, diseased cattle, badgers, and
other small mammals

Mode of Transmission
Spread by respiratory droplets
Direct invasion through mucous membranes

Incubation
4 to 12 weeks
Subsequent risk of pulmonary infection is greatest
within the first year
Infections may persist for a lifetime

Prevention
Education regarding the mode of transmission and
early diagnosis
Monitoring of groups at risk (people who are HIV-
positive, recent immigrants, homeless people,
people residing in crowded, substandard hous-
ing)
Report new cases
Implement AFB isolation immediately with any sus-
pected cases (see p. 49)
Eliminate tuberculosis among dairy cattle
Pasteurize milk

AN OVERVIEW OF COMMON INFECTIOUS DISEASES*†

AIDS
Transmission through blood and body fluids, sexual contact, sharing IV needles, contaminated blood, and from mother to fetus.

Considerations. Education regarding mode of transmission, avoidance of sexual contact with infected persons, use of latex condoms, proper blood screening of all transfusable products, and proper handling of needles and other contaminated material.

Chickenpox/Herpes Zoster Virus (Varicella/Shingles)
Transmission through respiratory droplets or by direct contact with open lesions.

Considerations. Strict isolation, avoidance of direct contact with lesions, and administration of varicella-zoster immune globulin. Caregivers should be chickenpox immune.

Chlamydia
Transmission through sexual contact.

Considerations. Public education, use of latex condoms.

German Measles (Rubella)
Transmission through respiratory droplets.

Considerations. Education regarding vaccines and prenatal care, avoidance of contact.

---

*Universal Precautions are required for all persons with infectious diseases.
†Check state requirements for reporting infectious diseases.

Gonorrhea

Transmission through vaginal secretions, semen, sexual contact.

Considerations. Public education regarding mode of transmission, use of latex condoms.

Hepatitis A

Transmission through direct contact with water, food, or feces.

Considerations. Hand washing before touching food, proper water and sewage treatment, reporting of cases, immunoglobulin vaccination when traveling to high-risk areas, proper disposal of contaminants.

Hepatitis B

Transmission through all fluids of an infected source.

Considerations. Hepatitis B vaccination, public education, blood screening, use of gloves when handling secretions, proper sterilization of equipment, reporting of all known cases to disease control centers.

Hepatitis C

Transmission through contaminated blood, plasma, and needles.

Considerations. See hepatitis B.

Influenza

Transmission through respiratory droplets.

Considerations. Public education about vaccines.

Measles (Red, Hard, Morbilli, Rubeola)

Transmission through airborne droplets or direct contact with lesions.

Considerations. Public education about vaccine, avoidance of contact with infected persons.

Meningitis (Bacterial)
Transmission through airborne droplets or direct contact.
Considerations. Public education, vaccination, early prophylaxis of exposed contacts.

Mononucleosis
Transmission through saliva.
Considerations. Public education, good hygiene.

Mumps
Transmission through airborne droplets and saliva.
Considerations. Vaccination.

Pneumonia
Transmission through airborne droplets.
Considerations. Vaccination, good hygiene.

Polio (Poliomyelitis)
Transmission through oral or fecal contact.
Considerations. Vaccination.

Salmonellosis
Transmission through ingestion of contaminated food.
Considerations. Proper cooking and storage of food, good hand washing prior to food preparation.

Syphilis
Transmission through sexual contact, direct contact with lesions, and blood transfusions.

Considerations. Public education regarding transmission, prenatal screening, and prenatal follow-up; use of latex condoms, blood screening.

Tetanus (Lockjaw)
Transmission through direct contact of wounds with infected soil or feces.
Considerations. Public education regarding mode of transmission, vaccination.

Tuberculosis
Transmission through airborne droplets; bovine TB through unpasteurized milk.
Considerations. Public education and screening, improvement of overcrowded living conditions, and pasteurization of milk.

Typhoid Fever
Transmission through contaminated water, urine, or feces.
Considerations. Good hygiene, sanitary water, proper sewage care, and vaccinations.

Whooping Cough (Pertussis)
Transmission through airborne droplets and nasal discharge.
Considerations. Vaccination, wearing of masks when near infected clients, reporting of all cases.

Specimen Collection Techniques

Amount Needed*	Collection Device*	Specimen Collection and Transport*
Wound Culture		
As much as possible (after cleaning skin to remove flora)	Cotton-tipped swab or syringe	Place clean test tube or culturette tube on clean paper towel. After swabbing center of wound site, grasp collection tube by holding it with paper towel. Carefully insert swab without touching outside of tube. After washing hands and securing tube's top, transfer labeled tube into bag for transport to laboratory.
Blood Culture		
10 ml per culture bottle, from two different veni-puncture sites (Volume may differ based on collection containers.)	Syringes and culture media bottles	Perform venipuncture at two different sites to decrease likelihood of both specimens being contaminated by skin flora. Inject 10 ml of blood into each bottle. Wash hands. Secure tops of bottles, label specimens, send to lab.

Stool Culture

Small amount, approximately size of a walnut

Clean cup with seal top (not necessary to be sterile) and tongue blade

Place cup on clean paper towel in client's bathroom. Using tongue blade, collect needed amount of feces from bedpan. Transfer feces to cup without touching cup's outside surface. Wash hands and place seal on cup. Transfer specimen cup into clean bag for transport to laboratory.

Urine Culture

1-5 ml

Syringe and sterile cup

Place cup or tube on clean towel in client's bathroom. Use syringe to collect specimen if client has Foley catheter. Have client follow procedure to obtain clean-voided specimen if not catheterized. Transfer urine into sterile container by injecting urine from syringe or pouring it from used container. Wash hands and secure top of labeled container. Transfer labeled specimen into clean bag for transport to laboratory.

From Potter PA, Perry AG: *Fundamentals of nursing*, ed 3, St. Louis, 1993, Mosby.
*Agency policies may differ on type of containers, amount of specimen material required, and bagging.

TYPES OF IMMUNITY

Active antibodies produced in body; long lasting
  Natural antibodies are produced during an active infection
    Examples chickenpox, mumps, measles
  Artificial vaccines of actual antigens
    Examples mumps, measles, rubella (MMR)
Passive antibodies produced outside the body; short acting
  Natural antibodies are passed from mother to child through placenta and breast milk
  Artificial injected immune serum

ANTIBODY FUNCTIONS

IgM first to respond; activates the complement system; stimulates ingestion by macrophage; principal antibody of the blood
IgG most prevalent antibody; major antibody of the tissues; produced after IgM; only antibody to cross placenta; antitoxin; antiviral
IgA principal antibody of the GI tract; found in tears, saliva, sweat, breast milk; protects epithelial lining
IgD only in minute concentrations; function unknown
IgE for allergic reactions

CHAPTER 4

Basic Nursing Assessments

For a more in-depth study of basic nursing assessments consult the following publications:

AJN/Mosby: *Nursing boards review for the NCLEX-RN examination,* ed 9, St Louis, 1993, Mosby.

Austrin MG, Austrin HR: *Learning medical terminology,* ed 7, St Louis, 1991, Mosby.

Phipps WJ, Long BC, Woods NF: *Medical-surgical nursing: concepts and clinical practice,* ed 4, St Louis, 1991, Mosby.

Potter PA: *Pocket guide to health assessment,* ed 3, St Louis, 1994, Mosby.

Potter PA, Perry AG: *Fundamentals of nursing: concepts, process, and practice,* ed 3, St Louis, 1993, Mosby.

THE CLIENT INTERVIEW

Demographics
Include name, address, sex, age, birth date, marital status or significant other, religion, race, education, occupation, hobbies, significant life events.

Past Health History
Includes history of smoking, heart disease, alcohol or other drug use or abuse, surgeries, injuries, childhood diseases and vaccinations, hypertension, diabetes, arthritis, seizures, cancer, emotional problems, transfusions, drug or food allergies, perception of client's health or illness, lifestyle, hygiene and eating habits, health practices.

Past Family Medical History
Includes history of heart disease, alcohol or drug use or abuse, diabetes, arthritis, cancer, emotional problems.

Current Situation
Reasons for seeking help or chief complaint include annual check-up, follow-up care, second opinion, new symptoms, monitoring existing health problem(s).

History of Present Illness
Includes location and quality of symptoms, chronology, aggravating and alleviating factors, associated symptoms, effect on lifestyle, measures used to deal with symptoms, review of body systems.

FUNCTIONAL ASSESSMENT

Health Perceptions
General health (good, fair, poor)
Tobacco/alcohol use (how much, how long)
Recreational or prescribed medications (list)
Hygiene practices

Nutrition
Type of diet (list)
Enjoys snacks (yes/no, what type)
Fluid intake (types of fluids)
Fluid restriction (yes/no)
Skin (normal, dry, rash)
Teeth (own, dentures, bridge)
Weight (recent gain or loss)

Respiration/Circulation
Respiratory problems (shortness of breath)
Smoking history
Circulation problems (chest pain, edema, pacemaker)

Elimination
Upper GI (nausea, vomiting, dysphagia, discomfort)
Bowels (frequency, consistency, last bowel movement, ostomy)
Bladder (incontinence, dysuria, urgency, frequency, nocturia, hematuria)

Activity/Exercise
Energy level (high, normal, low)
Usual exercise/activity patterns (recent changes)
Needs assistance with (eating, bathing, dressing)
Requirements (cane, walker, wheelchair, crutches)

Sleep

Problems (falling asleep, early waking, hours per night, napping)

Methods used to facilitate sleep

Feelings upon waking (fatigued, refreshed)

Cognitive

Educational level

Learning needs

Communication barriers (list)

Memory loss (yes/no)

Developmental age

Reads English (yes/no)

Other languages (list)

Sensory

Hearing/vision (no problems, impaired, devices)

Pain (yes/no, how managed)

Coping/Stress

Needs (social services, financial counselor)

May need (home care, nursing home)

Coping mechanisms used by client

Self-Perception

How illness/wellness is affecting patient

Body image or self-esteem concerns

Role/Relationships

Significant other or emergency contacts

Primary, secondary, or tertiary roles

Role changes caused by illness/wellness

Role conflicts caused by illness/wellness

Sexuality

Last menstrual period, menopause, breast examination

Testicular examination

How illness may affect sexuality

How hospitalization may affect sexuality

Any questions, needs, or additional concerns

Values/Beliefs

Religious or cultural affiliation

Religious or cultural beliefs concerning health or illness

Holiday or food restrictions while hospitalized

PHYSICAL ASSESSMENT

Appearance
Stage of development, general health, striking features, height, weight, behavior, posture, communication skills, grooming, hygiene

Skin
Color, consistency, temperature, turgor, integrity, texture, lesions, mucous membranes

Hair
Color, texture, amount, distribution

Nails
Color, texture, shape, size

Neurologic
Pupil reaction, motor and verbal responses, gait, reflexes, neurologic checks

Musculoskeletal
Range of motion, gait, tone, posture

Cardiovascular
Heart rate and rhythm, Homans' sign, peripheral pulses and temperature, edema

Respiratory
Rate, rhythm, depth, effort, quality, expansion, cough, breath sounds, sputum production, color, and amount, tracheostomy size, nasal patency

Gastrointestinal
Abdominal contour, bowel sounds, nausea, vomiting, ostomy type and care, fecal frequency, consistency, presence of blood

Genitourinary
Urine color, character, amount, odor, ostomy

Classification of Percussion Sounds			
Sounds	**Pitch**	**Duration**	**Example**
Flat	high	short	muscle
Dull	medium	medium	liver, heart
Resonant	low	long	lungs
Hyperresonant	lower	longer	emphysemic lungs
Tympanic	lowest	longest	stomach, colon

ASSESSMENT TECHNIQUES
Inspection by visual or auditory observation
Auscultation by listening to sounds using a stethoscope
Palpation by touching
  Fingertips: best for texture, moisture, shape
  Palmar surface of fingers: best for vibration
  Dorsum of hand: best for temperature
Percussion by striking the body and assessing the sound
  Light percussion: best for tenderness, density
  Sharp percussion: best for reflexes

TEMPERATURE

Normal Oral Averages:

	° C	° F
Infant:	36-38	97-100
Child:	37	98.6
Adult:	37	98.6
Elderly:	36	98

Time Required for Reading a Glass Thermometer

Oral: 3 to 5 minutes
Axillary: 9 to 10 minutes
Rectal: 2 to 4 minutes

Time Required for Reading an Electronic Thermometer

Hold the thermometer in place until the light or auditory signal indicates a reading

Time Required for Reading a Disposable Thermometer

Hold the thermometer in place until the chemically impregnated dots change color (about 45 seconds)

Time Required for Reading a Tympanic Thermometer

Hold the thermometer in place until the reading is displayed (about 2 seconds)

Distance of Insertion for Rectal Thermometer

Child:	1 inch
Adult:	1½ inches

Conversion Used for Fahrenheit

Axillary: Oral minus 1° F
Rectal: Oral plus 1° F

Special Factors

Circadian rhythm lower temperatures in A.M., higher in P.M.

Hormones progesterone will raise temperature

Emotions anxiety will raise temperature

Clinical Signs of Fever

Onset increased heart rate, increased respirations, pallor, cool skin, cyanosis, chills, decreased sweating, increased temperature

Course flushed, warm skin, increased heart rate and respiration, increased thirst, mild dehydration, drowsiness, restlessness, decreased appetite, weakness

Abatement flushed skin, decreased shivering, dehydration, diaphoresis

Fever Patterns

Fungal rises slowly and stays high

Intermittent spikes but falls to normal each day

Persistent either remains elevated or low grade; often caused by tumors of the central nervous system

Relapsing febrile for several days, alternating with normal temperatures; often caused by parasites or urinary tract infections

Remittent spikes and falls, but not to normal; often noted with abscesses, tuberculosis, or influenza viruses

Septic wide peak and nadir, often rigors and diaphoresis; often caused by gram-negative organisms

Sustained same as persistent

THERMAL DISORDERS

Hypothermia temperature under 34° C or 94° F
   Treatment: warm slowly

Frostbite constriction of vessels, numbness, pale
   skin
   Treatment: warm slowly

Hyperthermia any temperature above normal; severe hyperthermia is indicated by temperatures
   at or above 42.2° C or 108° F
   Treatment: replace fluids, watch for chilling

Heat stroke temperature above 42.2° C or 108° F
   Treatment: ice to groin and axilla

Heat cramps spasms of muscles
   Treatment: replace fluids, watch for chilling

Temperature Conversions

° F ° C	° F ° C	° F ° C
95.0-35.0	100.2-37.9	105.1-40.6
95.2-35.1	**100.4-38.0**	105.4-40.8
95.4-35.2	100.6-38.1	105.6-40.9
95.5-35.3	100.8-38.2	**105.8-41.0**
95.7-35.4	101.0-38.3	106.0-41.1
95.9-35.5	101.1-38.4	106.2-41.2
96.1-35.6	101.3-38.5	106.3-41.3
96.3-35.7	101.5-38.6	106.5-41.4
96.6-35.9	101.7-38.7	106.7-41.5
96.8-36.0	102.0-38.8	106.9-41.6
97.0-36.1	**102.2-39.0**	107.2-41.8
97.2-36.2	102.4-39.1	107.4-41.9
97.3-36.3	102.6-39.2	**107.6-42.0**
97.5-36.4	102.8-39.3	107.8-42.1
97.7-36.5	103.0-39.4	108.0-42.2
97.9-36.5	103.1-39.5	108.1-42.3
98.2-36.8	103.3-39.6	108.3-42.4
98.4-36.9	103.6-39.8	108.5-42.5
98.6-37.0	103.8-39.9	108.7-42.6
98.8-37.1	**104.0-40.0**	109.0-42.7
99.9-37.2	104.2-40.1	109.2-42.9
99.1-37.3	104.4-40.2	109.4-43.0
99.4-37.3	104.5-40.3	109.6-43.1
99.5-37.5	104.7-40.4	109.8-43.2
100.0-37.8	105.0-40.5	109.9-43.3

To convert to Fahrenheit: $F = (C \times \frac{9}{5}) + 32$
To convert to Celsius: $C = (F - 32) \times \frac{5}{9}$

PULSE

Normal Ranges With Averages

Infant: 90-(120)-160 beats per minute
Child: 80-(100)-120 beats per minute
Adult: Female: 60-(80)-100 beats per minute
        Male: 55-(75)-95 beats per minute

Assessments

Volume/Amplitude of Peripheral Pulses

0 = absent
1+ = weak/thready
2+ = normal
3+ = bounding

Rhythm

Regular normal
Regular/irregular usually regular but occasionally
  irregular
Bigeminal skips every other beat (monitor needed
  for detection)

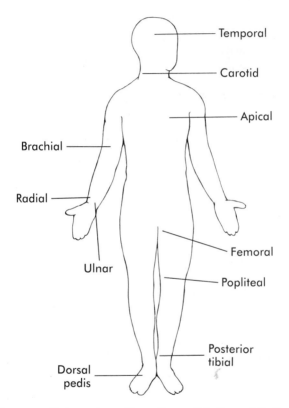

Figure 4-1 Pulse points. (From Potter PA, Perry AG: *Fundamentals of nursing,* ed 3, St Louis, 1993, Mosby.)

RESPIRATION

Normal Ranges
Infant: 30 to 80 respirations per minute
Child: 20 to 30 respirations per minute
Adult: 15 to 20 respirations per minute

Assessments
Depth: deep or shallow
Rhythm: even or uneven
Effort: ease, quiet, or with great effort
Expansion: symmetrical or asymmetrical
Cough: productive, nonproductive, or absent
Auscultation: clear, good air exchanged through-
out; adventitious; crackles, wheezes; diminished,
lowered, or distant sounds; absent, no sounds

BLOOD PRESSURE

Normal Averages
Newborn: 65-90/30-60
Infant: (1 year) 65-125/40-90
        (2 years) 75-100/40-90
Child: (4 years) 80-120/45-85
       (6 years) 85-115/50-60
Adolescent: (12 years) 95-135/50-70
            (16 years) 100-140/50-70
Adult: (18-60 years) 110-140/60-90
       (60+ years) 120-140/80-90

Orthostatic/Postural Changes
Take blood pressure and pulse with client lying
down. Then have client sit or stand for 1 minute.
Retake blood pressure and pulse. Record both sets
of numbers. If client is orthostatic, pressure will de-

crease (20-30 mm/Hg) and pulse will increase (5-25 beats per minute) when sitting or standing. Record and report any orthostasis.

Korotkoff Sounds

Sounds of Blood Pressure

Phase I: systole (sharp thud)
Phase II: systole (swishing sound)
Phase III: systole (low thud)
Phase IV: diastole (begins fading)
Phase V: diastole (silence)
Blood volume amount of blood in the system
Decreased blood volume equals decreased pressure, meaning increased need for fluids
Increased blood volume equals increased pressure, meaning need for less fluids
Cardiac output stroke volume multiplied by heart rate
Diastole ventricular relaxation
Pulse pressure systole minus diastole (normal range is 25 to 50)
Systole ventricular contraction
Viscosity thickness of the blood
Increased viscosity equals increased pressure meaning more work on the heart

The Cuff
· Cuff should be 20% wider than diameter of limb
· Too narrow a cuff leads to false high readings
· Too wide a cuff leads to false low readings
· Too loose a cuff leads to false high readings
· Deflating too slowly leads to false high diastolic readings
· Deflating too fast leads to false low systolic and high diastolic readings

HEIGHT AND WEIGHT CONVERSIONS

Height

Inch	Cm	Cm	Inch
1	2.5	1	0.4
2	5.1	2	0.8
4	10.2	3	1.2
6	15.2	4	1.6
8	20.3	5	2.0
10	25.4	6	2.4
20	50.8	8	3.1
30	76.2	10	3.9
40	101.6	20	7.9
50	127.0	30	11.8
60	152.4	40	15.7
70	177.8	50	19.7
80	203.2	60	23.6
90	227.6	70	27.6
100	254.0	80	31.5
150	381.0	90	35.4
200	508.0	100	39.4

1 inch =	1 cm =
2.54 cm	0.3937 inch

From Thompson JM, Bowers AC: *Health assessment: an illustrated pocket guide,* St Louis, 1992, Mosby.

Weight

LB	Kg	Kg	LB
1	0.5	1	2.2
2	0.9	2	4.4
4	1.8	3	6.6
6	2.7	4	8.8
8	3.6	5	11.0
10	4.5	6	13.2
20	9.1	8	17.6
30	13.6	10	22
40	18.2	20	44
50	22.7	30	66
60	27.3	40	88
70	31.8	50	110
80	36.4	60	132
90	40.9	70	154
100	45.4	80	176
150	66.2	90	198
200	90.8	100	220

1 lb =	1 kg =
0.454 kg	2.204 lb

From Thompson JM, Bowers AC: *Health assessment: an illustrated pocket guide,* St Louis, 1992, Mosby.

DESIRABLE WEIGHTS

Desirable Weights for Men
(According to Frame, Ages 25-59)

Height*		Weight†		
Feet	**Inches**	**Small Frame**	**Medium Frame**	**Large Frame**
5	2	128-134	131-141	138-150
5	3	130-136	133-143	140-153
5	4	132-138	135-145	142-156
5	5	134-140	137-148	144-160
5	6	136-142	139-151	146-164
5	7	138-145	142-154	149-168
5	8	140-148	145-157	152-172
5	9	142-151	148-160	155-176
5	10	144-154	151-163	158-180
5	11	146-157	154-166	161-184
6	0	149-160	157-170	164-188
6	1	152-164	160-174	168-192
6	2	155-168	164-178	172-197
6	3	158-172	167-182	176-202
6	4	162-176	171-187	181-207

Data from: Build study, 1979, Society of Actuaries and Association of Life Insurance Medical Directors of America, 1980.
Copyright 1983 Metropolitan Life Insurance Company.
*Shoes with 1-inch heels.
†Weight in pounds (in indoor clothing weighing 5 pounds).

Desirable Weights for Women
(According to Frame, Ages 25-59)

Height*		Weight†		
Feet	Inches	Small Frame	Medium Frame	Large Frame
4	10	102-111	109-121	118-131
4	11	103-113	111-123	120-134
5	0	104-114	113-126	122-137
5	1	106-118	115-129	125-140
5	2	108-121	118-132	128-143
5	3	111-123	121-135	131-147
5	4	114-127	124-138	134-151
5	5	117-130	127-141	137-155
5	6	120-133	130-144	140-159
5	7	123-136	133-147	143-163
5	8	126-139	136-150	146-167
5	9	129-142	139-153	149-170
5	10	132-145	142-156	152-173
5	11	135-148	145-159	155-176
6	0	138-151	148-162	158-179

Data from: Build study, 1979, Society of Actuaries and Association of Life Insurance Medical Directors of America, 1980.
Copyright 1983 Metropolitan Life Insurance Company.
*Shoes with 1-inch heels.
†Weight in pounds (in indoor clothing weighing 5 pounds).

Documentation

For a more in-depth study of documentation consult the following publications:

AJN/Mosby: *Nursing boards review for the NCLEX-RN examination,* ed 9, St Louis, 1993, Mosby.

Anderson KN, Anderson LE: *Mosby's pocket dictionary of medicine, nursing, and allied health,* St Louis, 1994, Mosby.

Austrin MG, Austrin HR: *Learning medical terminology,* ed 7, St Louis, 1991, Mosby.

Potter PA, Perry AG: *Fundamentals of nursing: concepts, process, and practice,* ed 3, St Louis, 1993, Mosby.

THE NURSING PROCESS

Assessment data collection; tools used include client and family interviews, functional areas, physical assessments, and laboratory tests; subjective aspects are those observed by client; objective aspects are those observed by nurse

Analysis interpretation of collected client data; determination of nursing diagnosis and plan of care; formation of nursing diagnoses

Planning formation of client's plan of care; client goals are outcomes to be achieved by client

Implementation nursing interventions; client's plan of care is based on assessments, analysis, and expected outcomes

Evaluation degree to which client's outcomes have been achieved; revision is an alteration in plan of care when expected outcomes are not achieved

NURSING DIAGNOSES BY FUNCTIONAL AREA

Health Perception
Growth and development, altered
Health maintenance, altered
Health seeking behavior (specify)
Injury, high risk for

Nutrition
Body temperature, altered, high risk for
Fluid volume deficit (1)
Fluid volume deficit (2)
Fluid volume deficit, high risk for
Fluid volume excess
Hyperthermia
Hypothermia
Infant feeding pattern, ineffective
Infection, high risk for
Nutrition, altered: less than body requirements
Nutrition, altered: more than body requirements
Nutrition, altered: high risk for more than body requirements
Oral mucous membrane, altered
Swallowing, impaired
Tissue integrity, impaired

Respiration/Circulation
Airway clearance, ineffective
Aspiration, high risk for
Breathing pattern, ineffective
Cardiac output, decreased
Gas exchange, impaired
Tissue perfusion, altered (specify type) (renal, cerebral, cardiopulmonary, gastrointestinal, peripheral)

Skin integrity, impaired
Skin integrity, impaired, high risk for
Ventilation, inability to sustain spontaneous
Ventilatory weaning process, dysfunctional

Elimination
Bowel incontinence
Constipation
Constipation, colonic
Constipation, perceived
Diarrhea
Incontinence, functional
Incontinence, reflex
Incontinence, stress
Incontinence, total
Incontinence, urge
Urinary elimination, altered
Urinary retention

Activity/Exercise
Activity intolerance
Activity intolerance, high risk for
Disuse syndrome
Diversional activity deficit
Fatigue
Home maintenance management, impaired
Mobility, impaired physical
Peripheral neurovascular dysfunction, high risk for
Self-care deficit, bathing/hygiene
Self-care deficit, dressing/grooming
Self-care deficit, feeding
Self-care deficit, toileting

Sleep
Sleep pattern disturbance

Cognition

Decisional conflict (specify)
Dysreflexia
Knowledge deficit (specify)
Pain
Pain, chronic
Sensory/perceptual alteration (specify) (visual, auditory, kinesthetic, gustatory, tactile, olfactory)
Thought process, altered

Coping/Stress

Adjustment, impaired
Anxiety
Coping, defensive
Coping, family: potential for growth
Coping, ineffective family: compromised
Coping, ineffective family: disabling
Coping, ineffective individual
Denial, ineffective
Fear
Management of therapeutic regimen (individuals), ineffective
Poisoning, high risk for
Post-trauma response
Rape-trauma syndrome
Rape-trauma syndrome: compound reaction
Rape-trauma syndrome: silent reaction
Relocation stress syndrome
Self-mutilation, high risk for
Suffocation, high risk for
Violence, high risk for: self-directed or directed at others

Self-Perception

Body image disturbance
Hopelessness

Personal identity disturbance
Powerlessness
Self-esteem disturbance
Self-esteem, chronic low
Self-esteem, situational low

Role/Relationships
Breastfeeding, effective
Breastfeeding, ineffective
Breastfeeding, interrupted
Caregiver role strain
Caregiver role strain, high risk for
Communication, impaired verbal
Family processes, altered
Grieving, anticipatory
Grieving, dysfunctional
Noncompliance (specify)
Parenting, altered
Parenting, altered, high risk for
Parental role conflict
Protection, altered
Role performance, altered
Social interaction, impaired
Social isolation
Trauma, high risk for
Unilateral neglect

Sexuality
Sexual dysfunction
Sexuality patterns, altered

Values/Beliefs
Spiritual distress (distress of the human spirit)

NANDA-APPROVED NURSING DIAGNOSES BY ALPHABETICAL LISTING

Activity intolerance
Activity intolerance, high risk for
Adjustment, impaired
Airway clearance, ineffective
Anxiety
Aspiration, high risk for
Body image disturbance
Body temperature, altered, high risk for
Bowel incontinence
Breastfeeding, effective
Breastfeeding, ineffective
Breastfeeding, interrupted
Breathing pattern, ineffective
Cardiac output, decreased
Caregiver role strain
Caregiver role strain, high risk for
Communication, impaired verbal
Constipation
Constipation, colonic
Constipation, perceived
Coping, defensive
Coping, family: potential for growth
Coping, ineffective family: compromised
Coping, ineffective family: disabling
Coping, ineffective individual
Decisional conflict (specify)
Denial, ineffective
Diarrhea
Disuse syndrome, high risk for
Diversional activity deficit
Dysreflexia
Family processes, altered
Fatigue

Fear
Fluid volume deficit (1)
Fluid volume deficit (2)
Fluid volume deficit, high risk for
Fluid volume excess
Gas exchange, impaired
Grieving, anticipatory
Grieving, dysfunctional
Growth and development, altered
Health maintenance, altered
Health-seeking behaviors (specify)
Home maintenance management, impaired
Hopelessness
Hyperthermia
Hypothermia
Incontinence, functional
Incontinence, reflex
Incontinence, stress
Incontinence, total
Incontinence, urge
Infant feeding pattern, ineffective
Infection, high risk for
Injury, high risk for
Knowledge deficit (specify)
Management of therapeutic regimen (individuals),
    ineffective
Mobility, impaired physical
Noncompliance (specify)
Nutrition: altered: less than body requirements
Nutrition, altered: more than body requirements
Nutrition, altered: high risk for more than body re-
    quirements
Oral mucous membrane, altered
Pain
Pain, chronic
Parental role conflict

Parenting, altered
Parenting, altered, high risk for
Peripheral neurovascular dysfunction, high risk for
Personal identity disturbance
Poisoning, high risk for
Post-trauma response
Powerlessness
Protection, altered
Rape-trauma syndrome
Rape-trauma syndrome: compound reaction
Rape-trauma syndrome: silent reaction
Relocation stress syndrome
Role performance, altered
Self-care deficit, bathing/hygiene
Self-care deficit, dressing/grooming
Self-care deficit, feeding
Self-care deficit, toileting
Self-esteem disturbance
Self-esteem, chronic low
Self-esteem, situational low
Self-mutilation, high risk for
Sensory/perceptual alterations (specify) (visual, auditory, kinesthetic, gustatory, tactile, olfactory)
Sexual dysfunction
Sexuality patterns, altered
Skin integrity, impaired
Skin integrity, impaired, high risk for
Sleep pattern disturbance
Social interaction, impaired
Social isolation
Spiritual distress (distress of the human spirit)
Suffocation, high risk for
Swallowing, impaired
Thermoregulation, ineffective
Thought processes, altered
Tissue integrity, impaired

Tissue perfusion, altered (specify type) (renal, cerebral, cardiopulmonary, gastrointestinal, peripheral)

Trauma, high risk for

Unilateral neglect

Urinary elimination, altered

Urinary retention

Ventilation, inability to sustain spontaneous

Ventilatory weaning process, dysfunctional

Violence, high risk for: self-directed or directed at others

DEVELOPING A CLIENT'S PLAN OF CARE

The components of the client's plan of care are based on the nursing process, beginning with the client history and assessments. The assessment information is the basis for developing the nursing diagnosis. The client outcomes or intended results are formed to give direction to the nursing interventions. The nursing interventions are the actions needed to achieve the desired client outcomes. The four parts of a care plan are shown on the opposite page.

INDIVIDUALIZING CARE PLANS

When developing a client care plan, the following considerations are needed in order to individualize the plan to meet each client's needs:

The client's age, gender, level of education, developmental level, general health status (current and prior to illness) disabilities (physical or mental), strength, and support systems.

Nursing Diagnosis	Client Outcome	Nursing Intervention	Evaluation
The Nursing Diagnosis			
List diagnosis	List the goals	List the interventions	—
Related to Specific problem	Each action should have an outcome	Actions per nurse	Can the client accomplish goals?
Secondary to Medical diagnosis	Consider the time needed to achieve the goals	Actions per client	Did the client accomplish goals?
As Manifested by List the signs/symptoms	Consider individualizing the care plan	Individualize interventions	Did symptoms resolve?

CRITICAL PATHWAYS

Critical pathways, part of managed care, incorporates a multidisciplinary approach to client care. When developing a client's plan of care through the use of critical pathways, consider some of the following questions:

Medicine

Which medical treatments will be recommended for the client? How will the medical treatments affect the plan of care and the client's outcomes? How will the prognosis affect the plan of care and the client's outcomes?

Pharmacy

What medications will be prescribed for the client? How will the medications affect the plan of care and the client's outcomes?

Therapy

Will physical or occupational therapy be prescribed for the client? How will physical or occupational therapy affect the plan of care and the client's outcomes?

Discharge Plans

What kind of discharge planning will the client need? When in the client's course of treatment should discharge planning begin? How will the discharge plans affect the plan of care and the client's outcomes?

Social Work

Will financial, social, or family services be needed for the client? How will these services affect the plan of care and the client's outcomes?

Chaplain

Will emotional or spiritual support be needed for the client? How will this support affect the plan of care and the client's outcomes?

CHARTING

Source-oriented records include admission sheet, physicians' orders, history, nurses' notes, tests, and reports

Problem-oriented records include data base, problem list, physicians' orders, care plans, and progress notes

Progress Notes

Examples include:

SOAP subjective data, objective data, assessment, plan

SOAPIE subjective, objective, assessment, plan, intervention, evaluation

AIR assessment, intervention, results

Narrative notes written in paragraph form

Flowsheet notes written in graph or checklist form

The Client's Chart is a Legal Document

- Be complete, concise, legible, and accurate.
- Use ink, sign all charting, cross out errors with a single line, and initial.
- Don't erase or use "white out." Don't leave spaces.
- Use only standard nursing abbreviations and proper medical terminology.
- Include date and time.
- Use proper grammar and accurate spelling.
- Documentation can be called as evidence in a legal action.

KARDEX

Includes:

Demographic information

List of medications and IV fluids

List of daily treatments, diagnostic tests, and laboratory tests

Allergies, problem list, activity, diet, and discharge plans

CHANGE OF SHIFT REPORT

Includes:

Client's name, age, room number, and diagnosis

Reason for admission, date and type of surgery if applicable

Significant changes during the last 24 hours

Tests and procedures during the last shift

Tests and procedures for the upcoming shift

Important laboratory data, current physical and emotional assessments

Vital signs if abnormal, intake and output, IV fluid status

Activity, discharge planning

Update changes or effectiveness of care plan on appropriate document

CHAPTER 6

Integumentary System

Common Integumentary Abnormalities
Common Skin Color Abnormalities
Abnormalities of the Nail Bed
Primary Skin Lesions
Secondary Skin Lesions
Pressure Points
Pressure Ulcer Stages
The Mouth

For a more in-depth study of the integumentary system
consult the following publications:

AJN/Mosby: *Nursing boards review for the NCLEX-RN examination,* ed 9,
   St Louis, 1993, Mosby.
Anderson KN, Anderson LE: *Mosby's pocket dictionary of medicine,
   nursing, and allied health,* St Louis, 1994, Mosby.
Austrin MG, Austrin HR: *Learning medical terminology,* ed 7, St Louis,
   1991, Mosby.
Phipps WJ, Long BC, Woods NF: *Medical-surgical nursing: concepts and
   clinical practice,* ed 4, St Louis, 1991, Mosby.
Potter PA, Perry AG: *Fundamentals of nursing: concepts, process, and
   practice,* ed 3, St Louis, 1993, Mosby.

COMMON INTEGUMENTARY ABNORMALITIES

Type	Characteristics	Assess for
Edema	fluid accumulation	trauma, murmur, third heart sound
Diaphoresis	sweating	pain, fever, anxiety, insulin reaction
Bromhidrosis	foul perspiration	infection, poor hygiene
Hirsutism	hair growth	adrenal function
Petechia	red/purple spots	hepatic function, drug reactions
Alopecia	hair loss	hypopituitarism, medications, fever, starvation

COMMON SKIN COLOR ABNORMALITIES

Type	Characteristics
Albinism	decreased pigmentation
Vitiligo	white patches on exposed areas
Mongolian spots	black and blue spots on back and buttocks
Jaundice	yellow pigmentation of skin or sclera
Ecchymosis	black and blue marks; assess for trauma, bleeding time, or hepatic function
Cyanosis	bluish color of lips, earlobes, or nail; assess lung and heart status

ABNORMALITIES OF THE NAIL BED

160 degrees — Normal nail: Approximately 160-degree angle between nail plate and nail

180 degrees — Clubbing: Change in angle between nail and nail base (eventually larger than 180 degrees); nail bed softening, with nail flattening; often enlargement of fingertips

180 degrees — *Causes:* Chronic lack of oxygen: heart or pulmonary disease

Beau's lines: Transverse depressions in nails indicating temporary disturbance of nail growth (Nail grows out over several months.)

Causes: Systemic illness such as severe infection, nail injury

Koilonychia (spoon nail): Concave curves

Causes: Iron deficiency anemia, syphilis, use of strong detergents

Splinter hemorrhages: Red or brown linear streaks in nail bed

Causes: Minor trauma, subacute bacterial endocarditis, trichinosis

Paronychia: Inflammation of skin at base of nail

Causes: Local infection, trauma

Figure 6-1 Abnormalities of the nail bed. (From Potter PA, Perry AG: *Fundamentals of nursing,* ed 3, St Louis, 1993, Mosby.)

PRIMARY SKIN LESIONS

Type	Definition	Example
Macule	flat, nonpalpable	freckle, measles
Papule	palpable, < 1 cm diameter	wart, psoriasis
Vesicle	palpable, < 1 cm, with fluid	blister, chickenpox
Nodule	hard, < 1 cm, into dermis	dermofibroma
Plaque	palpable or not, >1 cm	psoriasis, candidiasis
Bulla	vesicle, > 1 cm	poison oak, impetigo
Tumor	nodule, > 1 cm	lipoma, fibroma
Pustule	pus-filled vesicle	acne
Wheal	irregular, flat-topped	—
Cyst	fluid-filled, large	—

SECONDARY SKIN LESIONS

Type	Definition	Example
Scale	dead epithelium	psoriasis
Erosion	absence of epidermis	chancre
Crust	dried exudate	blister
Fissure	crack in the epidermis	cracked lips
Ulcer	necrotic epidermis	open sore
Scar	connective tissue	healing site
Keloid	overgrowth of scar	—
Licheni-fication	thickening of skin	eczema
Hyperke-ratosis	thickening of skin	callus

PRESSURE POINTS

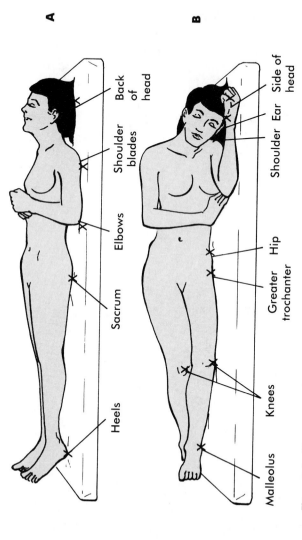

Figure 6-2 Pressure points. **A,** Supine position. **B,** Lateral position. (From Sorrentino SA: *Mosby's textbook for nursing assistants*, ed 3, St Louis, 1992, Mosby.)

Continued

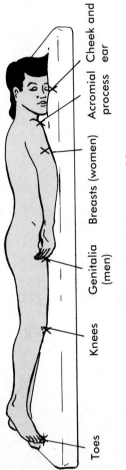

Figure 6-2, cont'd. C, Prone position.

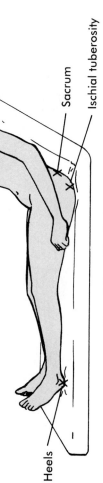

Figure 6-2, cont'd. D, Fowler's position.

Continued

E

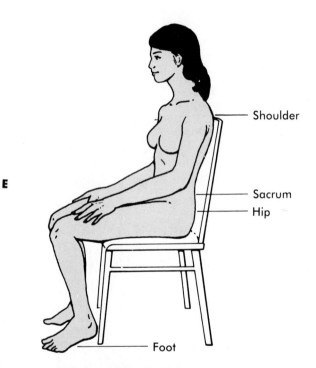

Figure 6-2, cont'd. **E,** Sitting position.

PRESSURE ULCER STAGES

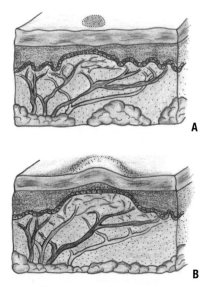

Figure 6-3 Pressure ulcer stages. **A,** Stage I. **B,** Stage II. (From Potter PA, Perry AG: *Fundamentals of nursing,* ed 3, St Louis, 1993, Mosby.) *Continued*

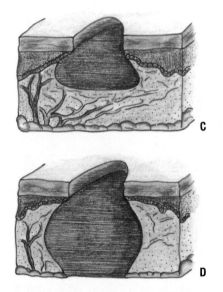

Figure 6-3, cont'd. **C,** Stage III. **D,** Stage IV.

The Mouth

Structure	Normal	Abnormal	Assess for
Lips	pinkish	pallor	anemia
	bluish (in black clients)	pallor	anemia
	smooth	blister	herpes
	symmetrical	swelling	allergic reaction
	moist	red; cracked	vitamin B deficiency
Bucca	pinkish	pallor	anemia; leukoplakia/cancer
	moist	dry	dehydration
Gums	pinkish	red; swollen	dilantin excess; leukemia; vitamin C deficiency
		dark lines	bismuth poisoning

Continued

The Mouth—cont'd

Structure	Normal	Abnormal	Assess for
Periodontium	pinkish	red; swollen	calcium deposits
Saliva	moderate	excessive	9th or 10th cranial nerve injury
Tongue	centered	not centered	12th cranial nerve damage
	dark pink	red; sore	anemia
		decreased papillae	riboflavin/niacin deficits
	smooth	vertical fissure	dehydration
	medium sized	oversized	hypothyroidism
Uvula	centered	not centered	tumor
	moves	doesn't move	9th or 10th cranial nerve damage
Tonsils	pink	red	pharyngitis
		swollen	tonsillitis

Skeletal System

For a more in-depth study of the skeletal system consult the following publications:

AJN/Mosby: *Nursing boards review for the NCLEX-RN examination,* ed 9, St Louis, 1993, Mosby.

Anderson KN, Anderson LE: *Mosby's pocket dictionary of medicine, nursing, and allied health,* St Louis, 1994, Mosby.

Austrin MG, Austrin HR: *Learning medical terminology,* ed 7, St Louis 1991, Mosby.

Phipps WJ, Long BC, Woods NF: *Medical-surgical nursing: concepts and clinical practice,* ed 4, St Louis 1991, Mosby.

Potter PA, Perry AG: *Fundamentals of nursing: concepts, process, and practice,* ed 3, St Louis, 1993, Mosby.

SKELETON—ANTERIOR VIEW

1 Cranium	16 Ulna
2 Orbit	17 Radius
3 Maxilla	18 Sacrum
4 Mandible	19 Greater trochanter
5 Clavicle	20 Carpals
6 Sternum	21 Metacarpals
7 Humerus	22 Phalanges
8 Xiphoid process	23 Femur
9 Costal cartilage	24 Patella
10 Vertebral column	25 Tibia
11 Innominate (hip)	26 Fibula
12 Ilium	27 Tarsals
13 Pubis	28 Metatarsals
14 Ischium	29 Phalanges
15 Lesser trochanter	

Figure 7-1 Skeleton—anterior view. (From Austrin MG, Austrin HR: *Learning medical terminology*, ed 7, St Louis, 1991, Mosby.)

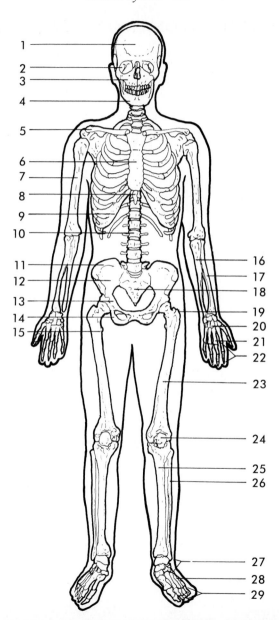

SKELETON—POSTERIOR VIEW

30	Acromion	39	Parietal bone
31	Scapula	40	Occipital bone
32	Humerus	41	Cervical vertebrae (7)
33	Olecranon	42	Thoracic vertebrae (12)
34	Radius	43	Lumbar vertebrae (5)
35	Ulna	44	Ilium
36	Femur	45	Sacrum
37	Fibula	46	Coccyx
38	Tibia	47	Ischium

Figure 7-2 Skeleton—posterior view. (From Austrin MG, Austrin HR: *Learning medical terminology,* ed 7, St Louis, 1991, Mosby.)

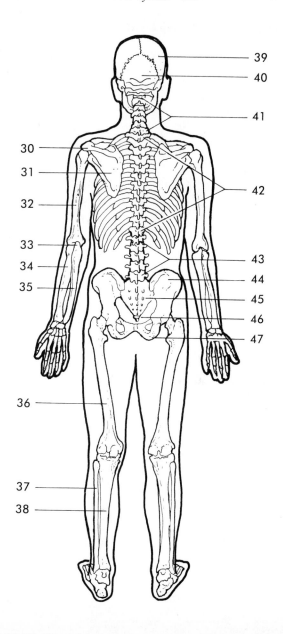

BONES OF THE SKULL

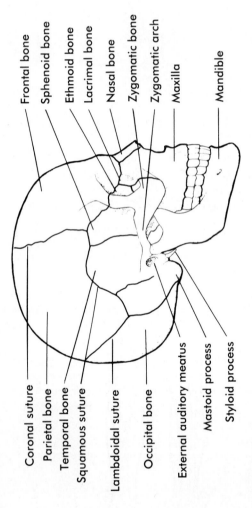

Figure 7-3   Bones and sutures of the skull. (From Austrin MG, Austrin HR: *Learning medical terminology*, ed 7, St Louis, 1991, Mosby.)

TYPES OF FRACTURES

Closed simple fracture does not break skin

Comminuted bone is splintered into fragments

Compression caused by compressive force; common in lumbar vertebrae

Depressed broken skull bone driven inward

Displaced fracture produces fragments that become misaligned

Greenstick fracture where one side of bone is broken and the other side is bent

Impacted telescoped bone is broken and wedged into another break

Incomplete continuity of the bone has not completely been destroyed

Longitudinal break runs parallel with the bone

Oblique fracture line runs at a 45-degree angle across the longitudinal axis

Open compound fracture breaks through skin (Can be categorized into grades 1 to 4 depending on severity)

Pathologic a disease process weakens bone structure so that a slight degree of trauma can cause fracture (Most common in osteoporosis and cancers of the bone)

Segmental fracture in two places (Also called double fracture)

Silver-fork fracture of lower end of radius

Spiral break coils around the bone; can be caused by a twisting force

Transverse fracture breaks across the bone at a 90-degree angle, along the longitudinal axis

POSSIBLE COMPLICATIONS FROM FRACTURES

Complications	Early Clinical Signs
Pulmonary embolism	substernal pain, dyspnea, rapid weak pulse; *may occur without symptoms*
Fat embolism	mental confusion, restlessness, fever, tachycardia, dyspnea
Gas gangrene	mental aberration, infection
Tetanus	tonic twitching, difficulty opening mouth; *may occur without symptoms*
Infection	pain, redness, swelling
Compartment syndrome	deep localized pain, numbness, weakness

TYPES OF TRACTION

Traction is a process whereby a steady pull is placed on a part or parts of the body. Traction can be used in reducing a fracture, maintaining a body position, immobilizing a limb, overcoming a muscle spasm, stretching an adhesion, and correcting deformities.

Countertraction a force that pulls against traction.

Suspension traction a process to suspend a body part using frames, splints, slings, ropes, pulleys, and weights.

Skin traction a process of applying wide bands directly to the skin and attaching weights to them (see Buck's and Russell's below).

Buck's traction a process of applying a straight pull on the affected extremity; used for muscle spasms and to immobilize a limb.

Russell's traction knee is suspended in a sling to which a rope is attached; allows for some movement and permits flexion of the knee joint; often used with a femur fracture.

Skeletal traction a process whereby traction is applied directly to the bone. A wire or pin is inserted through the bone, distal to the fracture.

TYPES OF SYNOVIAL JOINTS

Ball and socket head of one bone fits into socket of another bone; has greatest range of motion. Examples: hip and shoulder.

Hinge convex end of one bone fits into concave end of another bone; movement is on one plane; joints can flex or extend. Examples: elbow, knee, ankle, fingers, and toes.

Pivot arch-shaped; rotates only. Examples: C1 and C2 vertebrae.

Saddle convex bone fits into concave bone; movement is on two planes; joints can flex or extend and abduct or adduct. Example: thumb.

Gliding two flat bones move over each other. Examples: carpal, tarsal, clavicle, sternum, ribs, vertebrae, fibula, and tibia.

Condyloid oval-shaped; circular movement. Example: wrist.

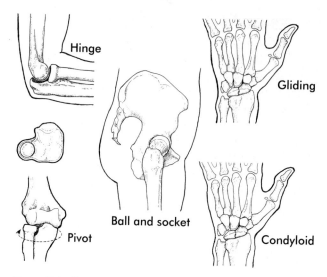

Figure 7-4 Synovial joints. (From Austrin MG, Austrin HR: *Learning medical terminology,* ed 7, St Louis, 1991, Mosby.)

CHAPTER 8

Muscular System

Anterior Superficial Muscles
Posterior Superficial Muscles
Anterior Facial Muscles
Lateral Facial Muscles
Grading Muscle Strength
Effects of Immobility
Range of Motion (ROM)
Use of Heat
Use of Cold
Giving a Massage
A Massage Technique
Positioning

For a more in-depth study of the muscular system consult
the following publications:

AJN/Mosby: *Nursing boards review for the NCLEX-RN examination,* ed 9,
      St Louis, 1993, Mosby.
Anderson KN, Anderson LE: *Mosby's pocket dictionary of medicine,
      nursing, and allied health,* St Louis, 1994, Mosby.
Austrin MG, Austrin HR: *Learning medical terminology,* ed 7, St Louis,
      1991, Mosby.
Phipps WJ, Long BC, Woods NF: *Medical-surgical nursing: concepts and
      clinical practice,* ed 4, St Louis, 1991, Mosby.
Potter PA, Perry AG: *Fundamentals of nursing: concepts, process, and
      practice,* ed 3, St Louis, 1993, Mosby.

ANTERIOR SUPERFICIAL MUSCLES

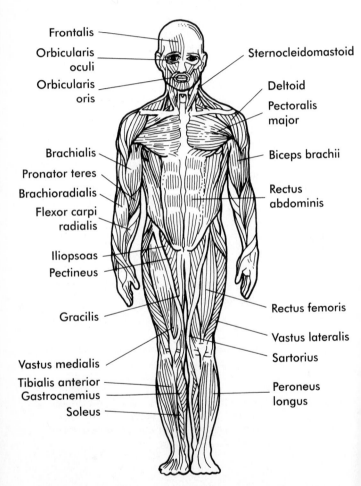

Figure 8-1 Anterior superficial muscles. (From Austrin MG, Austrin HR: *Learning medical terminology,* ed 7, St Louis, 1991, Mosby.)

POSTERIOR SUPERFICIAL MUSCLES

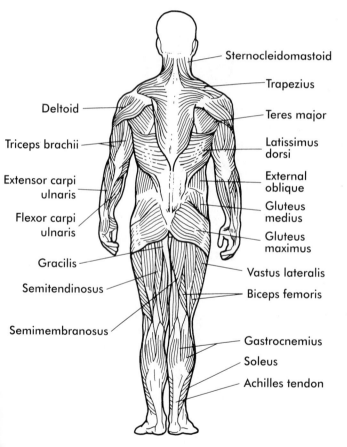

Figure 8-2 Posterior superficial muscles. (From Austrin MG, Austrin HR: *Learning medical terminology*, ed 7, St Louis, 1991, Mosby.)

ANTERIOR FACIAL MUSCLES

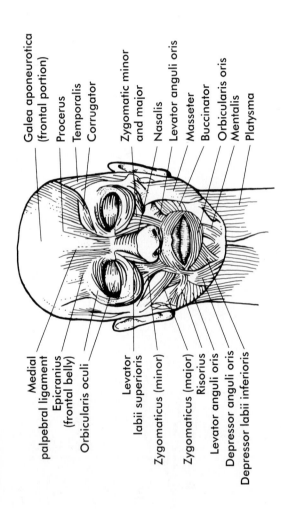

Figure 8-3 Anterior facial muscles. (From Austrin MG, Austrin HR: *Learning medical terminology*, ed 7, St Louis, 1991, Mosby.)

LATERAL FACIAL MUSCLES

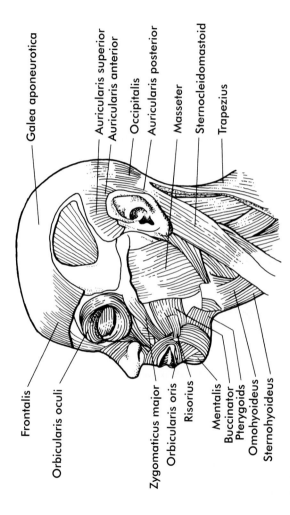

Figure 8-4 Lateral facial muscles. (From Austrin MG and Austrin HR: *Learning medical terminology*, ed 7, St Louis, 1991, Mosby.)

GRADING MUSCLE STRENGTH

Scale	Percent	Interpretation
5	100%	normal
4	75	full movement, but not against resistance
3	50	normal movement against gravity
2	25	movement if gravity eliminated
1	10	no movement
0	0	paralysis

EFFECTS OF IMMOBILITY

Benefits
Decreased need for oxygen.
Decreased metabolism and energy use.
Reduced pain.

Bowel Changes
Increased constipation caused by decreased peristalsis.
Poorer sphincter and abdominal muscle tone.

Cardiac Changes
Heart rate increase of one half beat per day, caused by increased sympathetic activity.
Decreased stroke volume and cardiac output caused by increased heart rate.
Hypotension caused by vasodilatation, leading to a thrombosis or edema.

Integumentary Changes
Decreased turgor caused by fluid shifts.
Increased decubitus ulcers caused by prolonged pressure.
Increased skin atrophy caused by decreased nutrition.

Metabolic Changes

Decreased metabolic rate.

Increased catabolism (protein breakdown) leading to a negative nitrogen imbalance, which results in poorer healing.

Hypoproteinemia leading to fluid shifts and edema.

Musculoskeletal Changes

Decreased muscle strength of 20% per week.

Decreased physical endurance and muscle mass.

Muscle atrophy caused by decreased contractions.

Osteoporosis caused by increased calcium extraction.

Demineralization begins on second day of immobilization.

Increased fractures caused by porous bones.

Increased hypercalcemia.

Muscle shortening leading to contracture.

Neurosensory Changes

Decreased tactile sensation.

Increased restlessness, drowsiness, and irritability.

Increased confusion and disorientation caused by hypercalcemia.

Respiratory Changes

Less alveoli expansion caused by less sighing.

Increased mucus in lungs caused by less ability to clear them.

Decreased chest movement restricts lung expansion.

Stiff intercostal muscles caused by less stretching.

Shallow respirations leading to decreased capacity.

Increased secretions caused by supine position of lungs.

Less oxygen leads to more carbon dioxide, which
results in acidosis.
Atelectasis caused by decreased blood flow.

Urinary Changes
Poor emptying caused by positioning.
Urinary stasis leads to more calcium in kidneys,
leading to increased renal calculi.
Urinary retention and distention caused by poor
emptying.
Incontinence caused by poor muscle tone.
Inability to void caused by overstretching of the
bladder.
Infection caused by stasis and alkalinity.
Urinary reflux caused by stasis, leading to infec-
tions.

Range of Motion (ROM)		
Type	**Function**	**Examples**
Flexion	decrease angle	bend elbow or knee, chin down, make fist, bend at waist or wrist, lift leg, bend toes
Extension	increase angle	straighten elbow or knee, chin straight, hands open, back, fingers, or toes straight
Hyperex-tension	straighten joint beyond limits	head tilted back, fingers pointed up
Abduction	move away from midline	legs or arms away from body, fingers spread apart
Adduction	move toward midline	legs together, arms at side, fingers together
Rotation	move around axis	circle of head, hand, foot, leg, arm, fingers, toes
Eversion	turn joint outward	foot or hand pointed away from the body
Inversion	turn joint inward	foot or hand pointed toward the body
Pronation	move joint down	palm downward, elbow inward
Supination	move joint up	palm upward, elbow outward

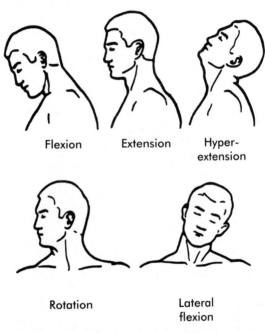

Flexion   Extension   Hyper-
                                 extension

Rotation   Lateral
                      flexion

Figure 8-5   Range-of-motion exercises. (From Sorrentino SA: *Mosby's textbook for nursing assistants,* ed 3, St Louis, 1992, Mosby.)

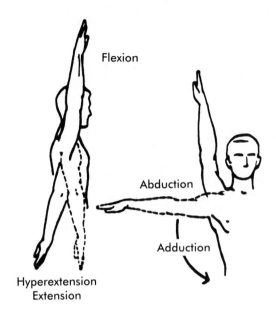

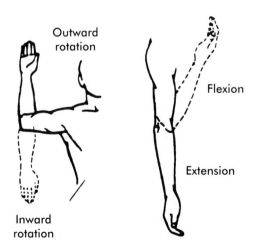

Figure 8-5, cont'd.

Continued

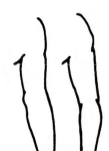

Supination   Pronation

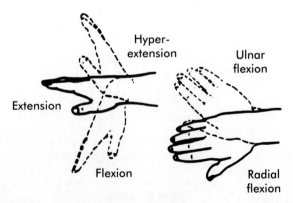

Figure 8-5, cont'd.

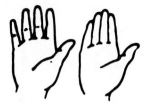

Abduction   Adduction

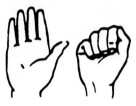

Extension   Flexion

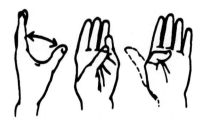

| Abduction Adduction | Opposition to little finger | Extension Flexion |

Figure 8-5, cont'd.

Continued

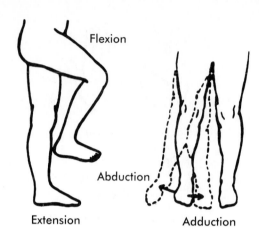

Flexion

Abduction

Extension

Adduction

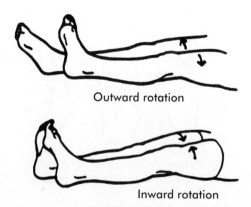

Outward rotation

Inward rotation

Figure 8-5, cont'd.

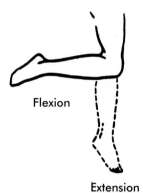

Flexion

Extension

Figure 8-5, cont'd.

Continued

Supination

Pronation

Abduction

Adduction

Extension

Flexion

Dorsal flexion

Plantar flexion

Figure 8-5, cont'd.

USE OF HEAT*

Local Effects
Increased skin temperature
Vasodilatation, which increases oxygen and nutrients to area
Increased muscle relaxation
Decreased stiffness and spasm
Increased peristalsis

Indications
Stiffness
Arthritis
Pain

Contraindications
Trauma because of increased bleeding
Edema because of increased fluid retention and edema
Malignant tumors because of increased cell growth
Burns because of increased cell damage
Open wounds because of increased bleeding
Acute areas such as appendix because of possible rupture
Testes because of destruction of sperm
Sensory-impaired clients because of increased chance of burns
Confused clients because of increased chance of injury

*The use of heat may require a physician's order.

USE OF COLD*

Local Effects
Vasoconstriction, which decreases oxygen to area
Decreased metabolism and thus decreased oxygen needs
Decreased fluid in area and thus decreased swelling
Decreased pain through numbness
Impaired circulation and increased cell death caused by lack of oxygen

Indications
Sprains
Fractures
Swelling
Bleeding

Contraindications
Open wounds because of decreased chance of healing
Impaired circulation because of increased chance of injury
Sensory-impaired clients because of increased chance of injury
Confused clients because of increased chance of injury

*The use of cold may require a physician's order.

GIVING A MASSAGE

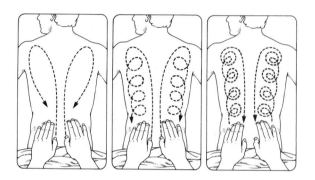

A MASSAGE TECHNIQUE
- Assess if a massage is contraindicated
- Start with the client lying flat or on his or her side
- Begin with the forehead and work down the body
- Use a gentle but firm touch
- Always stroke toward the heart
- Rub downward on the chest and back
- Stroke upward on the arms
- Use a light lotion or oil

POSITIONING

Dorsal lithotomy client lies on back with legs well apart. Knees are bent; stirrups are often used. Position is used to examine the bladder, vagina, rectum and perineum.

Dorsal recumbent client lies on back with legs slightly apart. Knees are slightly bent, with the soles of the feet flat on the bed.

Fowler's client is partly sitting with knees slightly bent. The head of the bed can be at semi-Fowler's (45 degrees) or high Fowler's (90 degrees).

Knee-chest client rests on knees and chest, with head turned to the side. Position is used to examine the rectum or vagina.

Left lateral client lies on left side, hips closer to the edge of the bed.

Left sims' client lies on left side, with right knee bent against the abdomen. Used in rectal exams and giving enemas.

Prone client lies on abdomen with arms at sides.

Reverse Trendelenburg client lies on back with legs together. Bed is straight, with head of bed higher than the foot.

Side lying client head is in straight line with spine. Use pillows to support head, arms, and upper leg.

Supine (**horizontal recumbent**) client lies on back with legs together and extended.

Trendelenburg client lies on back with legs together. Bed is straight, with head of bed lower then feet. Used in pelvic surgery.

Positions for Examination

Position	Areas Assessed	Rationale	Limitations
Sitting	Head and neck, back, posterior thorax and lungs, anterior thorax and lungs, breasts, axillae, heart, vital signs, and upper extremities	Sitting upright provides full expansion of lungs and provides better visualization of symmetry of upper body parts.	Physically weakened client may be unable to sit. Examiner should use supine position with head of bed elevated instead.

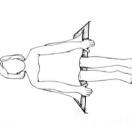

Continued

From Potter PA, Perry AG: *Fundamentals of nursing*, ed 3, St Louis, 1993, Mosby.

Positions for Examination—cont'd

Position	Areas Assessed	Rationale	Limitations
Supine	Head and neck, anterior thorax and lungs, breasts, axillae, heart, abdomen, extremities, pulses	This is most normally relaxed position. It prevents contracture of abdominal muscles and provides easy access to pulse sites.	If client becomes short of breath easily, examiner may need to raise head of bed.
Dorsal recumbent	Head and neck, anterior thorax and lungs, breasts, axillae, heart	Clients with painful disorders are more comfortable with kenes flexed.	Position is not used for abdominal assessment because it promotes contracture of abdominal muscles.

Positions for Examination—cont'd

Position	Areas Assessed	Rationale	Limitations
Lithotomy	Female genitalia and genital tract	This position provides maximal exposure of genitalia and facilitates insertion of vaginal speculum.	Lithotomy position is embarrassing and uncomfortable, so examiner minimizes time that client spends in it. Client is kept well draped. Client with severe arthritis or other joint deformity may be unable to assume this position.

Continued

Positions for Examination—cont'd

Position	Areas Assessed	Rationale	Limitations
Sims'	Rectum and vagina	Flexion of hip and knee improves exposure of rectal area.	Joint deformities may hinder client's ability to bend hip and knee.
Prone	Musculoskeletal system	This position is used only to assess extension of hip joint.	This position is intolerable for client with respiratory difficulties.
Knee-chest	Rectum	This position provides maximal exposure of rectal area.	This position is embarrassing and uncomfortable. Clients with arthritis or other joint deformities may be unable to assume this position.

CHAPTER 9

Nervous System

For a more in-depth study of the nervous system consult the following publications:

Phipps WJ, Long BC, Woods NF: *Medical-surgical nursing: concepts and clinical practice,* ed 4, St Louis, 1991, Mosby.
Potter PA, Perry AG: *Fundamentals of nursing: concepts, process, and practice,* ed 3, St Louis, 1993, Mosby.

STRUCTURES OF THE BRAIN

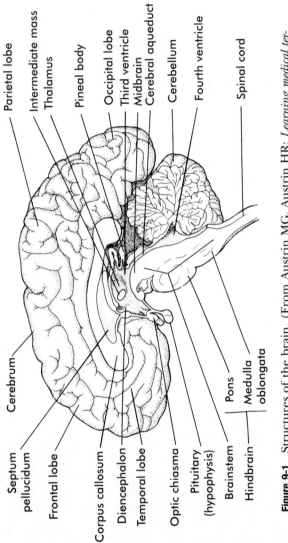

Figure 9-1 Structures of the brain. (From Austrin MG, Austrin HR: *Learning medical terminology*, ed 7, St Louis, 1991, Mosby.)

LEVELS OF CONSCIOUSNESS

Alert awake and aware, responds appropriately, begins conversation (A&O × 3: alert and oriented to person, place, time).

Lethargic sleeps but easily aroused, speaks and responds slowly but appropriately.

Obtunded difficult to arouse, slow to respond, and returns to sleep quickly.

Stuporous aroused only through pain; no verbal response, never fully awake.

Semicomatose responds only to pain but has gag and blink reflexes.

Comatose no response to pain; no reflexes or muscle tone.

NEUROLOGIC FUNCTION

Cerebral

Includes mental status, thought processes, emotions, level of consciousness, orientation, memory, language, appropriateness, intelligence, and developmental age.

Cranial Nerves

(See page 149.)

Cerebellar

Includes coordination and balance; muscle size, strength, and tone (see page 122); and evaluation of reflexes.

Glasgow Coma Scale		
Best eye opening response (Record "C" if eyes closed by swelling)	Spontaneously	4
	To speech	3
	To pain	2
	No response	1
Best motor response to painful stimuli (Record best upper limb response)	Obeys verbal command	6
	Localizes pain	5
	Flexion-withdrawal	4
	Flexion-abnormal	3
	Extension-abnormal	2
	No response	1
Best verbal response (Record "E" if endotracheal tube in place. "T" is tracheostomy tube in place)	Oriented × 3	5
	Conversation confused	4
	Speech inappropriate	3
	Sounds incomprehensible	2
	No response	1

Modified from Thompson JM, Bowers AC: *Health assessment: an illustrated pocket guide,* St Louis, 1992, Mosby.

A CLIENT'S SLEEP HISTORY
- Have the client describe his or her specific problem.
- Have the client describe his or her symptoms and alleviating factors.
- Assess the client's normal sleep pattern.
- Assess the client's normal bedtime rituals.
- Assess for current or recent physical illnesses.
- Assess for current or recent emotional stress.
- Assess for possible sleep disorders.
- Assess the client's current medications and their possible effects on sleep.

SLEEP DISORDERS
Bruxism tooth grinding during sleep

Insomnia chronic difficulty with sleep patterns

   Initial insomnia difficulty falling asleep

   Intermittent insomnia difficulty remaining asleep

   Terminal insomnia difficulty going back to sleep

Narcolepsy difficulty in regulating between sleep and awake states; person may fall asleep without warning

Nocturnal enuresis bedwetting

Sleep apnea intermittent periods of cessation of breathing during sleep

Sleep deprivation decrease in the amount and quality of sleep

Somnambulism sleepwalking, night terrors, or nightmares

Drugs and Their Effects on Sleep

Hypnotics

- Interfere with reaching deeper sleep stages
- Provide only temporary (1-week) increase in quantity of sleep
- Eventually cause "hangover" during day: excess drowsiness, confusion, decreased energy
- May worsen sleep apnea in older adults

Diuretics

- Cause nocturia

Antidepressants and Stimulants

- Suppress REM sleep

Alcohol

- Speeds onset of sleep
- Disrupts REM sleep
- Awakens person during night and causes difficulty returning to sleep

From Potter PA, Perry AG: *Fundamentals of nursing,* ed 3, St Louis, 1993, Mosby.

Drugs and Their Effects on Sleep—cont'd

Caffeine

- Prevents person from falling asleep
- May cause person to awaken during night

Digoxin

- Causes nightmares

Beta-Blockers

- Causes nightmares
- Causes insomnia
- Causes awakening from sleep

Valium

- Decreases stages 2, 4, and REM sleep
- Decreases awakenings

Narcotics (Morphine/Demerol)

- Suppress REM sleep
- If discontinued quickly, can increase risk of cardiac dysrhythmias because of "rebound REM" periods
- Cause increased awakenings and drowsiness

PERIPHERAL NERVES

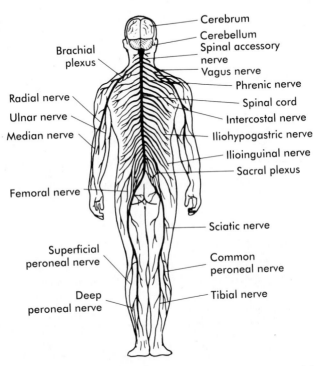

Figure 9-2 Peripheral nervous system, with some cranial nerves. (From Austrin MG, Austrin HR: *Learning medical terminology,* ed 7, St Louis, 1991, Mosby.)

Cranial Nerves

Number	Name	Type	Function	Method of Assessment
I	Olfactory	Sensory	Smell	ID odors
II	Optic	Sensory	Vision	Snellen's chart
III	Oculomotor	Motor	Vision	Pupil reaction
IV	Trochlear	Motor	Vision	Vertical vision
V	Trigeminal	Sensory	Cornea	Blink reflex
		Motor	Chewing	Clench teeth
VI	Abducens	Motor	Vision	Lateral vision
VII	Facial	Sensory	Taste	ID tastes
		Motor	Expression	Smile/frown
VIII	Acoustic	Sensory	Equilibrium	Weber's and Rinne tests
IX	Glossopharyngeal	Sensory	Taste	ID tastes
		Motor	Swallows	Gag reflex
X	Vagus	Sensory	Pharynx	ID tastes
		Motor	Vocal	Voice tones
XI	Accessory	Motor	Shoulders	Shrug shoulders
XII	Hypoglossal	Motor	Tongue	Protruding tongue

Types of Reflexes

Name	Elicited By	Response
Babinski	Stroking lateral sole of foot	Great toe fans out
Chaddock	Stroking below lateral malleolus	Great toe fans out
Oppenheim	Stroking tibial surface	Great toe fans out
Gordon	Squeezing calf muscle	Great toe fans out
Hoffmann	Flicking middle finger down	Flexion of the thumb
Ankle clonus	Brisk dorsiflexion of foot with knee flexed	Up and down movement of the foot
Kernig	Straightening leg with thigh flexed	Pain along posterior of thigh
Brudzinski	Flexing chin or chest	Limitations with pain

REFLEX GRADING SCALE

Grade	Symbols	Interpretation
5	5+	hyperactive (with clonus)
4	4+	hyperactive (very brisk)
3	3+	brisk
2	2+	normal (average)
1	1+	diminished but present
0	0	absent

PAIN ASSESSMENT
Gather information on the following areas:

Definition
The words used by the client to describe their pain, such as pressure, stabbing, sharp, tingling, dull, heavy, or cold. *It is important to use and understand the client's language concerning pain, and to believe the client who reports pain.*

Onset
When did the pain first begin (date and time)?

Duration
How long does the pain last (persistent, minutes to hours, comes and goes, seconds)? Does the pain occur at the same time each day?

Location
In what area of the body does the pain begin? It may be helpful to have the client point to the exact area if possible. NOTE: A client may say the pain is in the stomach but may point over lower abdominal area. Also ask if the pain radiates, moves, or goes to a different area of the body. Have the client point to these areas as well.

Severity
How bad is the pain? Or have the client rate the pain. Have a rating scale ready to use and explain your scale. Use the same scale in subsequent assessments. Examples: A zero to ten scale with zero being no pain and ten being the worst pain or color scale with blue being no pain and red being the worst pain.

Precipitating Factors

What was the client doing before the pain began (exercise, bending over, work)?

Aggravating Factors

What makes the pain worse?

Alleviating Factors

What makes the pain get better or go away (pain medications, relaxation, rest, music)?

PAIN RATING SCALES

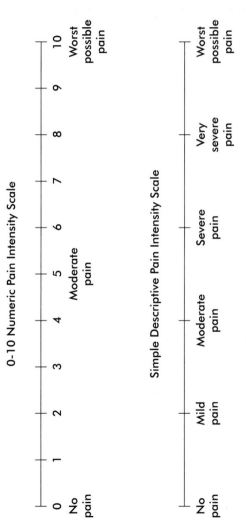

Figure 9-3 Pain rating scales.

NONPHARMACOLOGIC TREATMENTS OF PAIN

Biofeedback clients can learn to control muscle tension in order to reduce pain with the use of biofeedback units.

Cold used to decrease pain or swelling. (See p. 134.)

Distraction turning the client's attention to something other than the pain, such as music, visitors, or scenery.

Heat used to decrease tension. (See p. 133.)

Imagery employs the client's imagination to create pleasant mental pictures. These pictures are a form of distraction. This activity is said to be a form of self-hypnosis.

Massage (See p. 135.)

Menthol used to increase blood circulation to painful areas.

Nerve blocks used to block severe, unrelieved pain. A local anesthetic, sometimes combined with cortisone, is injected into or around a nerve.

Positioning (See p. 136.)

Pressure used to stimulate blood flow to painful areas. Apply firm but not excess pressure for 10 to 60 seconds.

Range of motion exercises (See p. 126.)

Relaxation relieves pain by reducing muscle tension. Music or relaxation tapes may be helpful.

TENS transcutaneous electric nerve stimulation. A mild electric current is thought to interrupt pain impulses.

Vibration used to stimulate blood flow to painful areas.

CHRONIC NONMALIGNANT PAIN: NURSING CARE GUIDELINES

Do not argue with the client about whether or not the client is in pain.

Do not refer to the client as a narcotics addict.

Do not tell the client that he or she will become an addict if he or she continues to receive narcotics.

Do not use a placebo to try to determine if the client has "real" pain.

Be alert to any changes in the client's pain condition or pain regiment.

Recognize the differences between acute and chronic pain.

Avoid sudden withdrawal of narcotics or sedatives from a client with chronic pain.

When analgesics are required give them orally if possible. (The effects of oral analgesics will generally last longer than IV or IM medications.)

Review analgesics being used for relief of chronic versus acute pain.

Offer pain relief alternatives. (See p. 154.)

Review the client's support systems and suggest additional ones if appropriate.

Help those living with the client to understand the client's pain management routine.

Assess the client for depression, anxiety, and stress. (Additional stresses may add to the client's overall pain experience.)

Assess suicidal risk.

Modified from McCaffery M, Beebe A: *Pain: clinical manual for nursing practice,* St. Louis, 1989, Mosby.

Average Adult Doses For Analgesics				
Drug	**IM Dose (MG)**	**Oral Dose (MG)**	**Half Life (HR)**	**Duration (HR)**
Aspirin	—	500-1000	30 min	4-6
Acetaminophen	—	500-1000	2-3	4-6
Ibuprofen	—	400-800	2-3	4-6
Salicylate	—	1000	1-4	6-12
Naproxen	—	500	2-3	6-8
Indomethacin	—	25	2-4	8-12
Ketorolac	30-60	—	2-3	6
Oxycodone (Percocet)	15-30	—	2-3	6
Propoxyphene (Darvon)	—	5	2-3	4-6
Levorphanol	—	30-65	1-2	4-6
Morphine	2	2-4	2-4	4-8
Codeine	2-15	10-60	1-3	3-7
Hydromorphone (Dilaudid)	25-60	15-60	2-4	4-6
Meperidine (Demerol)	1-4	1-10	1-2	4-5
Methadone	10-100	50-100	1-2	2-4
	10	5-40	1-3	4-6

THE EYE

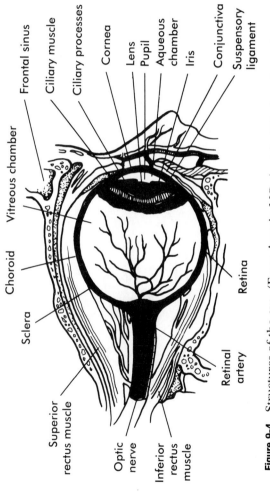

Figure 9-4 Structures of the eye. (From Austrin MG, Austrin HR: *Learning medical terminology,* ed 7, St Louis, 1991, Mosby.)

Continued

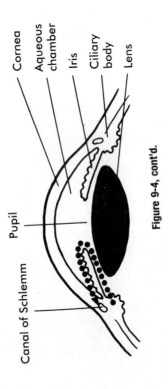

Figure 9-4, cont'd.

Contact Lens Care

Do

- Wash and rinse hands thoroughly before handling a lens.
- Keep fingernails clean.
- Remove lenses from their storage case one at a time and place on the eye.
- Start with the same lens (left or right) each time of insertion.
- Use lens placement technique learned from eye specialist.
- Use proper lens care products.
- Wear lenses daily and follow the prescribed wearing schedule.
- Remove a lens if it becomes uncomfortable.
- Keep regular appointments with the eye specialist.
- Remove lenses during sunbathing, showering, or swimming.

Do Not

- Use soaps that contain cream or perfume for cleansing lenses.
- Let fingernails touch lenses.
- Mix up lenses.
- Exceed prescribed wearing time.
- Use saliva to wet lenses.
- Use homemade saline solution or tap water to wet or clean lenses.
- Borrow or mix lens care solution

From Potter PA, Perry AG: *Fundamentals of nursing*, ed 3, St Louis, 1993, Mosby.

BRAILLE ALPHABET

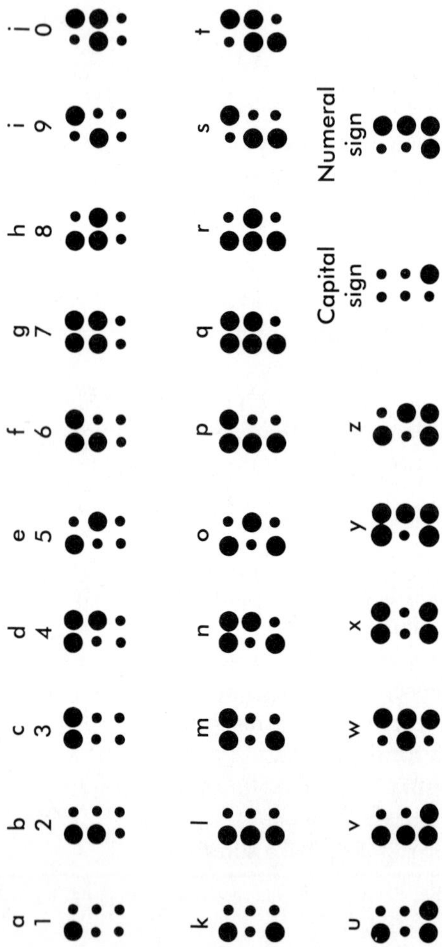

Figure 9-5 Braille alphabet. (From Sorrentino SA: *Mosby's textbook for nursing assistants,* ed 3, St Louis, 1992, Mosby.)

THE EAR

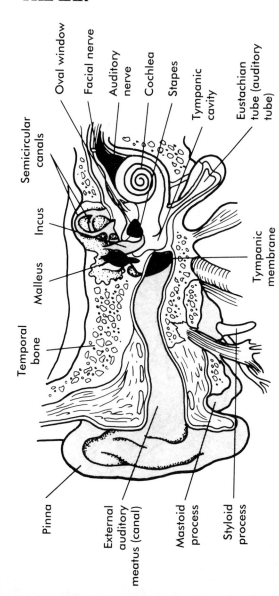

Figure 9-6 Structures of the ear. (From Austrin MG, Austrin HR: *Learning medical terminology*, ed 7, St Louis, 1991, Mosby.)

Assessing Client's Use of Sensory Aids

Eyeglasses

- Purpose for wearing glasses (e.g., reading, distance, or both)
- Methods used to clean glasses
- Presence of symptoms (e.g., blurred vision, photophobia, headaches, irritation)

Contact Lenses

- Type of lens worn
- Frequency and duration of time lenses are worn (including sleep time)
- Presence of symptoms (e.g., burning, excess tearing, redness, irritation, swelling, sensitivity to light)
- Techniques used by the client to cleanse, store, insert, and remove lenses
- Use of eyedrops or ointments
- Use of emergency identification bracelet or card that warns others to remove client's lenses in case of emergency

Artificial Eye

- Method used to insert and remove eye
- Method for cleansing eye
- Presence of symptoms (e.g., drainage, inflammation, pain involving the orbit)

Hearing Aid

- Type of aid worn
- Methods used to cleanse aid
- Client's ability to change battery and adjust hearing-aid volume

From Potter PA, Perry AG: *Fundamentals of nursing*, ed 3, St Louis, 1993, Mosby.

SIGN LANGUAGE

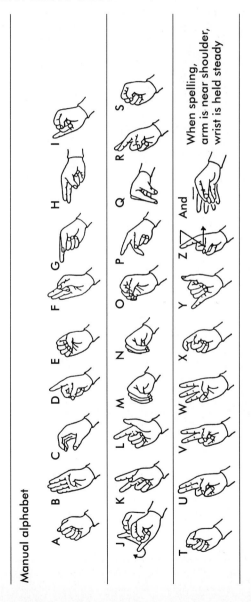

Figure 9-7 Sign language alphabet.

Continued

Numbers

Figure 9-7, cont'd. Sign language numbers.

CHAPTER 10

Circulatory System

Principal Arteries of the Body
Principal Veins of the Body
Circulation of Blood Through the Heart
Basic Cardiac Assessment
Cardiac History
Abnormal Heart Sounds
Pulse Grading Scale
Assessment of Pulse Sites
Quality and Pitch of Murmurs
Murmur Grading Scale
Edema Grading Scale
Tissue Perfusion

For a more in-depth study of the circulatory system consult
the following publications:

Anderson KN, Anderson LE: *Mosby's pocket dictionary of medicine,
nursing, and allied health,* St Louis, 1994, Mosby.
Austrin MG, Austrin HR: *Learning medical terminology,* St Louis, ed 7,
1991, Mosby.
Guzzetta CE, Dossey BM: *Cardiovascular nursing: holistic practice,* St
Louis, 1992, Mosby.
Phipps WJ, Long BC, Woods NF: *Medical-surgical nursing: concepts and
clinical practice,* ed 4, St Louis, 1991, Mosby.
Potter PA, Perry AG: *Fundamentals of nursing: concepts, process, and
practice,* ed 3, St Louis, 1993, Mosby.

PRINCIPAL ARTERIES OF THE BODY

1 Angular
2 Right common carotid
3 Brachiocephalic
4 Arch of aorta
5 Right coronary
6 Left coronary
7 Aorta
8 Celiac
9 Superior mesenteric
10 Common iliac
11 Internal iliac (hypogastric)
12 External iliac
13 Deep medial circumflex femoral
14 Deep femoral
15 Femoral
16 Popliteal
17 Anterior tibial
18 Peroneal
19 Posterior tibial
20 Dorsal pedis
21 Arcuate
22 Dorsal metatarsal
23 Occipital
24 Internal carotid
25 External carotid
26 Left common carotid
27 Subclavian
28 Pulmonary
29 Lateral thoracic
30 Axillary
31 Brachial
32 Splenic
33 Renal
34 Inferior mesenteric
35 Radial
36 Ulnar
37 Deep palmar arch
38 Superficial palmar arch
39 Digital

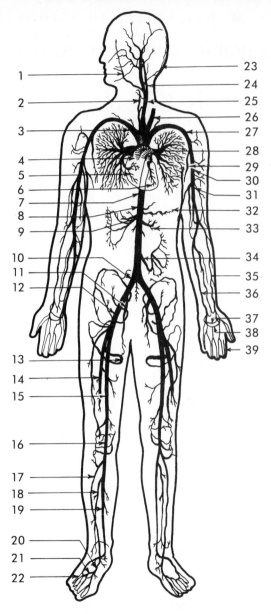

Figure 10-1 Principal arteries of the body. (From Austrin MG, Austrin HR: *Learning medical terminology*, ed 7, St Louis, 1991, Mosby.)

PRINCIPAL VEINS OF THE BODY

1 Angular
2 Anterior facial
3 Internal jugular
4 Right brachiocephalic
5 Subclavian
6 Superior vena cava
7 Right pulmonary
8 Right coronary
9 Inferior vena cava
10 Hepatic
11 Portal
12 Superior mesenteric
13 Common iliac
14 Superior sagittal sinus
15 Inferior sagittal sinus
16 Straight sinus
17 Transverse sinus
18 Cervical plexus
19 External jugular
20 Left brachiocephalic
21 Left pulmonary
22 Cephalic
23 Axillary
24 Left coronary
25 Basilic
26 Splenic
27 Median basilic
28 Long thoracic
29 Inferior mesenteric
30 Internal iliac (hypogastric)
31 External iliac
32 Volar digital
33 Femoral
34 Great saphenous
35 Popliteal
36 Peroneal
37 Posterior tibial
38 Anterior tibial
39 Dorsal venous arch

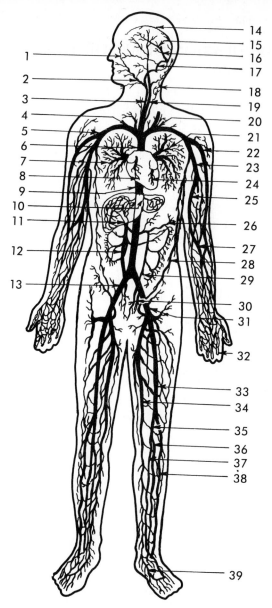

Figure 10-2 Principal veins of the body. (From Austrin MG, Austrin HR: *Learning medical terminology*, ed 7, St Louis, 1991, Mosby.)

CIRCULATION OF BLOOD THROUGH THE HEART

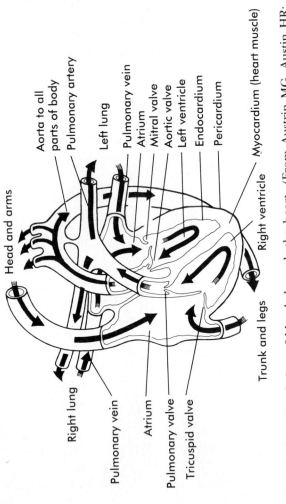

Figure 10-3 Circulation of blood through the heart. (From Austrin MG, Austin HR: *Learning medical terminology*, ed 7, St Louis, 1991, Mosby.)

BASIC CARDIAC ASSESSMENT

S1

First heart sound—heard when the mitral and tricuspid valves close. After ventricles are filled with blood a dull, low-pitched "lub" is heard. Systole begins when ventricles contract. Systole is shorter than diastole.

S2

Second heart sound—heard when the aortic and pulmonic valves close. After blood goes to aorta and pulmonary artery a high-pitched, snappy "dub" is heard.

CARDIAC HISTORY

Client History

Past heart attacks, rheumatic fever, fevers, hypertension, dizziness, syncope, diabetes, lung or endocrine diseases.

Health Habits

Smoking, alcohol, diet, exercise, stress.

Family History

Coronary disease, strokes, or obesity in parents or grandparents.

Signs and Symptoms

Chest pain, shortness of breath, orthopnea, syncope, hypertension, dyspnea, edema, cough, palpitations, wheezing, need for extra pillow to sleep, fatigue, weakness.

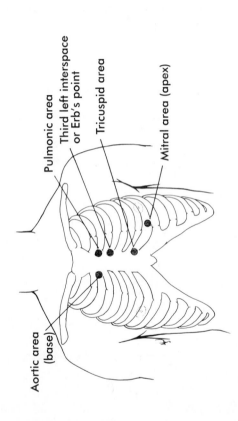

Figure 10-4 Topographic areas for cardiac auscultation. (From Phipps WJ, Long BC, Woods NF: *Medical-surgical nursing: concepts and clinical practice*, ed 4, St Louis, 1991, Mosby.)

ABNORMAL HEART SOUNDS

S1 varying intensity with different beats—indicates possible heart blockage.

S2 increased intensity at aortic valve—indicates possible hypertension

S3 increased intensity at pulmonic valve—indicates possible hypertension

Systole sharp sound—indicates possible deformity

Diastole presence of S3 in the elderly—indicates possible heart failure

S1 S2 S3 = "Ken tuck ky" S4 S1 S2 = "Ten nes see"

PULSE GRADING SCALE

4-Point Scale

0 no pulse
1+ weak, thready, fading, easily obliterated
2+ difficult to palpate
3+ normal
4+ bounding

3 Point Scale

0 absent
1+ weak, thready
2+ normal
3+ full, bounding

ASSESSMENT OF PULSE SITES

Temporal found over the **temporal bone,** above and lateral to the eye; easily accessible, used often in children.

Apical best found between the **fourth and fifth intercostal space,** midclavicular line; used to auscultate heart sounds, and before the administration of digoxin.

Carotid found on either side of the neck over the **carotid artery;** used to assess circulation during shock or cardiac arrest, and when other peripheral pulses are poor

Brachial found in the **antecubital area** of the arm; used to auscultate blood pressure and to assess circulation of the lower arm.

Radial found on the **thumb side of the forearm** at the wrist; used to assess circulation of the hand and peripheral circulation.

Ulnar found at the **wrist on the opposite side of the radius;** used to assess circulation of the hand and in Allen's assessment test.

Femoral found below the **inguinal ligament,** midway between the symphysis pubis and the anterosuperior iliac spine; used to assess circulation of the leg; can be used to assess circulation during shock or a cardiac arrest, or when other peripheral pulses are poor

Popliteal found **behind the knee;** used to assess lower leg circulation.

Posterior tibial found on the **inner side of each ankle;** used to assess foot circulation.

Dorsalis pedis found along the **top of the foot** between extension tendons of the great and first toes; used to assess the circulation of the foot.

QUALITY AND PITCH OF MURMURS

Type	Quality	Pitch
Aortic and pulmonary stenosis	Harsh	Medium-high
Mitral and tricuspid regurgitation	Blowing	High
Ventricular septal defect	Usually harsh	High
Mitral stenosis	Rumbling	Low
Aortic regurgitation	Blowing	High

MURMUR GRADING SCALE

1 difficult to hear
2 faint but recognizable
3 heard easily with stethoscope
4 loud, often with a palpable thrill
5 very loud; associated with a thrill
6 stethoscope not needed to hear; can be heard with stethoscope 1 inch from chest

EDEMA GRADING SCALE

1+ barely detectable
2+ indentation of <5 mm
3+ indentation of 5 to 10 mm
4+ indentation of >10 mm

Tissue Perfusion		
Area	**Abnormality**	**Assessment**
Skin Color	Cyanotic	Decreased venous return
	Pallor	Decreased arterial flow
	Dusky	Decreased arterial flow
Temperature	Cool	Decreased arterial flow
Fluid	Mild edema	Decreased arterial flow
	Great edema	Decreased venous return
Texture	Thin or thick	Decreased venous return and arterial flow
	Shiny	Decreased venous return and arterial flow
Nails	Cyanotic	Decreased arterial flow

CHAPTER 11

Respiratory System

For a more in-depth study of the respiratory system consult the following publications:

Anderson KN, Anderson LE: *Mosby's pocket dictionary of medicine, nursing, and allied health,* St Louis, 1994, Mosby.

Austrin MG, Austrin HR: *Learning medical terminology,* ed 7, St Louis, 1991, Mosby.

Guzzetta CE, Dossey BM: *Cardiovascular nursing: holistic practice,* St Louis, 1992, Mosby.

Phipps WJ, Long BC, Woods NF: *Medical-surgical nursing: concepts and clinical practice,* ed 4, St Louis, 1991, Mosby.

Potter PA, Perry AG: *Fundamentals of nursing: concepts, process, and practice,* ed 3, St Louis, 1993, Mosby.

LOWER RESPIRATORY TRACT

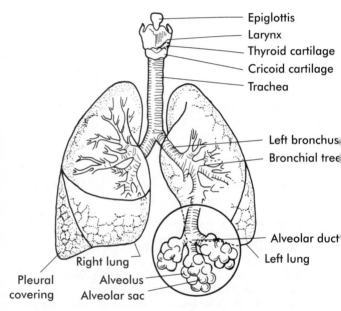

Figure 11-1 Lower respiratory tract. (From Austrin MG, Austrin HR: *Learning medical terminology,* ed 7, St Louis, 1991, Mosby.)

UPPER RESPIRATORY TRACT

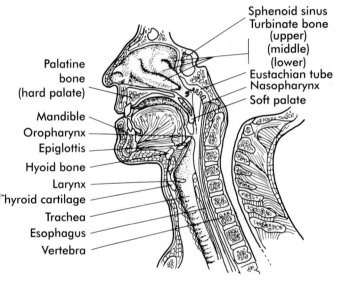

Figure 11-2 Upper respiratory tract. (From Austrin MG, Austrin HR: *Learning medical terminology,* ed 7, St Louis, 1991, Mosby.)

CHEST WALL LANDMARKS

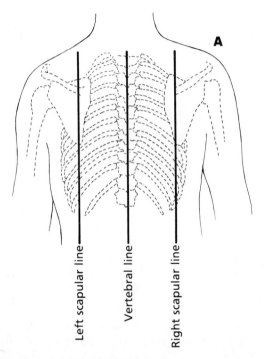

Figure 11-3 Chest wall landmarks. (From Potter PA, Perry AG *Fundamentals of nursing,* ed 3, St Louis, 1993, Mosby.)

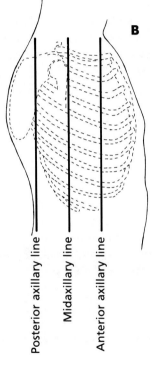

Posterior axillary line

Midaxillary line

Anterior axillary line

Figure 11-3, cont'd.

Continued

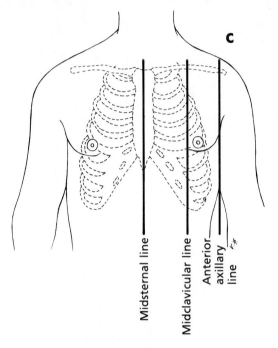

Fig. 11-3, cont'd.

NORMAL BREATH SOUNDS

Vesicular soft, low-pitched sighing over bronchiole and alveoli bases on inspiration.

Bronchial moderate, high pitched over trachea.

Bronchovesicular moderate sound over first and second intercostal space.

Trachea loudest and highest pitched of normal breath sounds, harsh and tubular.

Common Abnormalities of the Lung

Type	Characteristics	Assess for
Apnea	Periods of not breathing	Sleep problem, impending death
Bradypnea	<10 breaths per minute	Drug overdose, alcohol overdose
Dyspnea	Difficulty breathing	Low Hgb, acidosis
Stridor	High-pitched sounds	Obstruction
Tachypnea	>20 breaths per minute	Anxiety, fever
Hyperpnea	Increased rate and depth	Pain, reaction to altitude
Hyperventilation	Increased rate and depth	Acidosis
Cheyne-Stokes breathing	Alternating periods of hyperpnea and apnea	Impending death
Kussmaul respirations	Extreme rate and depth	Diabetic ketoacidosis, renal failure
Asymmetric	Lungs do not expand equally	Fractured ribs, missing lung, pneumothorax

ABNORMAL AND ADVENTITIOUS SOUNDS

Crackles/Rales fine, crackle-like sounds, usually on inspiration.

Alveolar high pitched
Bronchial low pitched

Rhonchi coarse, harsh, over fluid (usually on expiration).

Wheezes squeaky, musical on inspiration or expiration.

Friction Rub grating sound of pleurae rubbing together, generally on the anterior side.

COMMON LUNG DISORDERS

Asthma

Signs and Symptoms. Dyspnea, cough, tachypnea.
Listen for. Decreased sounds with wheezes.

Atelectasis

Signs and Symptoms. Tachypnea, cyanosis, use of accessory muscles.
Listen for. Decreased sound with crackles.

Bronchitis

Signs and Symptoms. Cough with sputum, sore throat and fever, prolonged expiration.
Listen for. prolonged expiration, wheezes, crackles.

Emphysema

Signs and Symptoms. Dyspnea, cough with sputum.
Listen for. Wheezes, rhonchi.

Neoplasm

Signs and Symptoms. Cough with sputum, possible chest pain.
Listen for. Decreased sounds.

Pleural Effusion

Signs and Symptoms. Pain, dyspnea, pallor, fever, cough.
Listen for. Decreased sounds, friction rub.

Pneumonia

Signs and Symptoms. Chills, productive cough, rapid swallow rate.
Listen for. Fine crackles or friction rub.

Pneumothorax

Signs and Symptoms. Pain, dyspnea, cyanosis, tachypnea.
Listen for. Decreased sound on affected side.

Pulmonary Edema

Signs and Symptoms. Tachypnea, cough, cyanosis, orthopnea, use of accessory muscles.
Listen for. Rales, rhonchi, wheezes.

Positions for Postural Drainage

Lung Segment	Position of Client
Adult	
Bilateral	High Fowler's

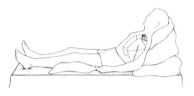

Apical segments	Sitting on side of bed
Right upper lobe— anterior segment	Supine with head elevated

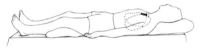

Left upper lobe— anterior segment	Supine with head elevated

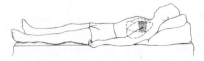

Modified from Potter PA, Perry AG: *Fundamentals of nursing,* St Louis, 1993, Mosby.

Positions for Postural Drainage—cont'd

Lung Segment	Position of Client
Right upper lobe— posterior segment	Side lying with right side of chest elevated on pillows

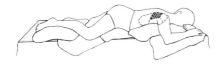

Left upper lobe— posterior segment	Side lying with left side of chest elevated on pillows

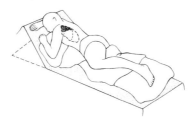

Right middle lobe— anterior segment	Three-fourths supine position with dependent lung in Trendelenburg position

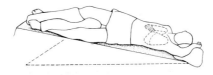

Continued.

Positions for Postural Drainage—cont'd

Lung Segment	Position of Client
Right middle lobe—posterior segment	Prone with thorax and abdomen elevated

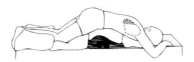

Both lower lobes—anterior segments	Supine in Trendelenburg

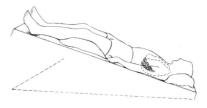

Left lower lobe—lateral segment	Right side lying in Trendelenburg position

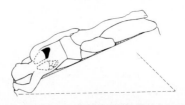

Positions for Postural Drainage—cont'd

Lung Segment	Position of Client
Right lower lobe—lateral segment	Left side lying in Trendelenburg position

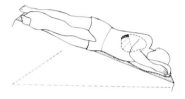

Right lower lobe—posterior segment	Prone with right side of chest elevated in Trendelenburg position

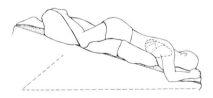

Both lower lobes—posterior segment	Prone in Trendelenburg position

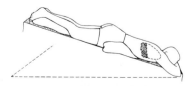

Continued.

Positions for Postural Drainage—cont'd

Lung Segment	Position of Client

Child

Bilateral—apical
  segments

Sitting on nurse's lap,
  leaning slightly for-
  ward flexed over pillow

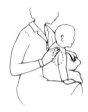

Bilateral—middle
  anterior segments

Sitting on nurse's lap,
  leaning against nurse

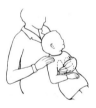

Bilateral lobes—
  anterior segments

Lying supine on nurse's
  lap, back supported
  with pillow

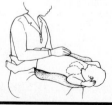

OXYGEN THERAPY*

Cannula
1 liter = 24% oxygen
2 liters = 28% oxygen
3 liters = 32% oxygen
4 liters = 36% oxygen
5 liters = 40% oxygen
6 liters = 44% oxygen

If client requires oxygen greater than 6 liters a mask may be needed. Humidification may be added for comfort.

Simple Mask
5-6 liters = 40% oxygen
7-8 liters = 50% oxygen
10 liters = 60% oxygen

Should not be run below 5 liters per minute

Partial Rebreathing Mask
6-10 liters = up to 80% oxygen

Level of oxygen will depend on client's overall respiratory and health status. *Should not be run below 5 liters per minute Reservoir bag should never be fully collapsed.*

Nonbreathing Mask
Will deliver 80%-100% oxygen. *Should not be run below 5 liters per minute. Reservoir bag should never be fully collapsed.*

---

*Oxygen is a drug and therefore a physician's order is required for use.

CHAPTER 12

Endocrine System

For a more in-depth study of the endocrine system consult the following publications:

AJN/Mosby: *Nursing boards review for the NCLEX-RN examination,* ed 9, St Louis, 1993, Mosby.

Anderson KN, Anderson LE: *Mosby's pocket dictionary of medicine, nursing, and allied health,* St Louis, 1994, Mosby.

Austrin MG, Austrin HR: *Learning medical terminology,* ed 7, St Louis, 1991, Mosby.

Phipps WJ, Long BC, Woods NF: *Medical-surgical nursing: concepts and clinical practice,* ed 4, St Louis, 1991, Mosby.

Potter PA, Perry AG: *Fundamentals of nursing: concepts, process, and practice,* ed 3, St Louis, 1993, Mosby.

ENDOCRINE GLANDS AND ASSOCIATED STRUCTURES

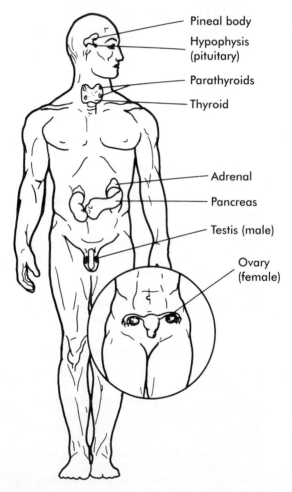

Figure 12-1 Endocrine glands. (From Austrin MG, Austrin HR: *Learning medical terminology,* ed 7, St Louis, 1991, Mosby.)

DIABETES

Type I (IDDM) Juvenile Onset	Type II (NIDDM) Adult Onset
Clinical Information	
10%-15% of diabetic cases	85%-90% of diabetic cases
Abrupt onset	Gradual onset
Autoimmune islet-cell destruction	Insulin resistance or deficiency
Generally begins before age 40 but can occur at any age	Generally begins after age 40 but can occur earlier
Clinical Manifestations	
Weight loss, increased hunger,	Fatigue, drowsiness
Excessive thirst, increased urinary frequency,	Blurred vision
Possible ketoacidosis	No ketoacidosis
Prone to ketosis	No ketosis
No endogenous insulin	Has endogenous insulin
Diet very important	Diet very important
Insulin mandatory	Insulin needed in 25% of cases
Oral hypoglycemic not used	Oral hypoglycemic used in 40% of cases

BLOOD GLUCOSE REACTIONS

Insulin Reaction Hypoglycemia Glucose level <60 mg/dl	**Diabetic Ketoacidosis** Hyperglycemia Glucose level >250 mg/dl
Clinical Manifestations	
Causes	
Too much insulin	Too little insulin
Skipped or delayed meals	Overeating
Too much exercise	Emotional stress, illness, infection, surgery, heart attack, stroke, pregnancy
Early Symptoms	
Sweatiness, shakiness, weakness	Excessive thirst
Headache, dizziness	Frequent urination
Hunger	Fatigue, weakness
Late Symptoms	
Numbness of lips/tongue	Abdominal pain, nausea, vomiting
Difficulty concentrating	General aches, loss of appetite
Mood change/irritability	Flushed, dry skin
Vision changes, pallor	Fruity breath, drowsiness
If Not Treated	
Seizures, coma	Labored breathing, coma

TREATMENT FOR BLOOD GLUCOSE REACTIONS

Insulin Reaction Hypoglycemia Glucose level <60 mg/dl	Diabetic Ketoacidosis Hyperglycemia Glucose level >250 mg/dl
One of the Following:	**All of the following:**
10-15 g glucose or 2 glucose tablets	Alert physician
5 pieces of candy or 4 oz juice	Monitor blood sugar
1 mg IM Glucagon	Test urine for ketones
Repeat any *one* of the above in 15 minutes if needed	Provide IV hydration per physician's orders
Document reaction	Provide potassium replacements
Inform physician	*Give insulin per physician's order*
	Document actions

REACTION PREVENTION TIPS

Insulin Reaction	Diabetic Ketoacidosis
Eat meals at same time each day	Follow prescribed eating schedule
If meals are delayed: For 1 hour: Drink 4 oz fruit juice For more than 2 hours: Eat 4 oz protein	Know factors that can raise blood sugar Avoid stress or overwork
Take correct insulin as scheduled	Take correct insulin as scheduled
Wear diabetic identification	Wear diabetic identification
Check blood sugar as needed	On sick days: *Do Not Stop Insulin* Check urine for ketones every 12 hours Monitor blood glucose every 2-4 hours Maintain good fluid intake Alert physician if glucose is >240 mg/dl
Carry a quick-acting sugar at all times	

General Client and Family Information

With an increase in activity, never omit insulin.

Before vacations call physician to see if insulin dose needs adjusting.

Know insulin peaks and how body reacts to insulin highs and lows.

Inform family and friends of possible reactions and how to treat them.

Hypoglycemic Agents

Types		Peak (Hours)	Duration (Hours)
Oral Agents	Chlorpropamide (Diabinese)	3-6	24-48
	Tolbutamide (Orinase)	5-8	6-12
	Tolazamide (Tolinase)	10	12-24
	Glipizide (Glucotrol)	1-3	12-24
	Glyburide (Diabeta, Micronase)	2-8	24
Insulin	Rapid Acting (onset 1 hour)		
	Crystalline zinc	2-4	5-8
	Regular	2-4	4-6
	Insulin zinc (Semilente)	6-10	12-16
	Regular human (Humulin-R, Novolin-R)	1-3	3-5

Hypoglycemic Agents—cont'd		
Types	**Peak (Hours)**	**Duration (Hours)**
Insulin—cont'd		
Intermediate Acting (onset 2-4 hours)		
Globin zinc (Iletin)	6-10	18-24
Isophane suspension (NPH)	8-12	18-24
Insulin suspension (Iletin Lente)	8-12	18-24
NPH human ispohane (Humulin-R, Novolin-R)	8-12	26-30
Long Acting (onset 4-6 hours)		
Protamine zinc (PZ)	16-24	24-36
Insulin extended (Ultralente)	16-24	more than 36
Lente human	16-24	24-30

Modified from AJN/Mosby: *Nursing boards review for the NCLEX-RN examination*, ed 9, St Louis, 1993, Mosby.

ADRENAL GLANDS

Cushing's Syndrome Hyperfunction	Addison's Disease Hypofunction
Clinical Manifestations	
Excessive cortisol production	Inadequate cortisol production
Increased ACTH from pituitary	Insufficient ACTH from pituitary
Increased protein catabolism	Flaccid muscles/paralysis
Muscle wasting and fragile skin	Muscle weakness and anorexia
Osteoporosis and compression fractures	Nausea/vomiting and diarrhea
Bruises easily/poor healing	Abdominal pain
Obesity/moon face/buffalo hump	Weight loss
Hyperglycemia and worsening of diabetes	Frequent hypoglycemia
Decreased immunity	Decreased cardiac output
Sodium and water retention	Hyponatremia and hypoosmolality
Edema/hypertension	Hypotension and dyshythmias
Hypokalemia/hypochloremia	Hyperkalemia
Renal calculi/hypercalcemia	Hypercalcemia
Irritability	Lethargy
Anxiety	Depression

PITUITARY GLAND*

Hyperpituitarism

Clinical Information

This disorder is generally caused by tumors, which lead to an increase in hormone levels. The most common hormones involved are:

GH growth hormone, which causes gigantism

ACTH adrenocorticotropic hormone, which causes Cushing's disease

TSH thyroid-stimulating hormone, which causes hyperthyroidism

LH luteinizing hormone

FSH follicle-stimulating hormone

Hypopituitarism

Clinical Information

This disorder is usually caused by tumors, necrosis, or glandular, dysfunction, leading to a decrease in hormone levels. The most common problems associated with hypopituitarism are:

Dwarfism caused by a decreased growth hormone

Hypophysectomy the removal or destruction of pituitary gland

Postpartum necrosis caused by hypotension after delivery

Functional disorders caused by starvation or anemia

*Specific problems, signs, and symptoms will depend on the hormone involved.

THYROID GLAND

Hyperthyroidism	Hypothyroidism
Clinical Manifestations	
Increased body metabolism	Decreased body metabolism
Nervousness/restlessness	Lethargy and headaches
Short attention span	Memory deficit
Tachycardia (>100 beats/min; bounding heart sounds)	Bradycardia (<60 beats/min; weak heart sounds)
Increased blood pressure	Decreased blood pressure
Reduced vital capacity	Lowered respiratory rate
Skin warm, moist and smooth	Skin cool, dry and rough
Hair fine, nails soft	Hair coarse, nails brittle
Weakness and fatigue	Weakness and fatigue
Demineralization of bones	Stiff joints
Hypercalcemia	Mild proteinuria
Brisk reflexes	Decreased reflexes
Increased appetite/weight loss	Decreased appetite/weight gain
Muscle wasting	Muscular stiffness
Diabetes worsens	Diabetic clients need less insulin
Increased stools	Constipation
Increased libido	Decreased libido
Decreased fertility	Decreased fertility
Higher body temperature	Lower body temperature

CHAPTER 13

Digestive System

For a more in-depth study of the digestive system consult the following publications:

AJN/Mosby: *Nursing boards review for the NCLEX-RN examination,* ed 9, St Louis, 1993, Mosby.

Anderson KN, Anderson LE: *Mosby's pocket dictionary of medicine, nursing, and allied health,* St Louis, 1994, Mosby.

Austrin MG, Austrin HR: *Learning medical terminology,* ed 7, St Louis, 1991, Mosby.

Phipps WJ, Long, BC, Woods NF: *Medical-surgical nursing: concepts and clinical practice,* ed 4, St Louis, 1991, Mosby.

Potter PA, Perry AG: *Fundamentals of nursing: concepts, process, and practice,* ed 3, St Louis, 1993, Mosby.

Williams, SR: *Nutrition and diet therapy,* ed 7, St Louis, 1993, Mosby.

DIGESTIVE SYSTEM AND ASSOCIATED STRUCTURES

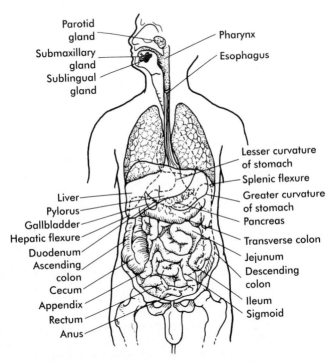

Figure 13-1 Digestive system and associated structure. (From Austrin MG, Austrin HR: *Learning medical terminology,* ed 7, St Louis, 1991, Mosby.)

Types of Diets

Type	Description	Client Complaint
Regular	Has all essentials, no restrictions	No special diet needed
Clear Liquid	Broth, tea, clear soda, strained juices, gelatin	Recovery from surgery or very ill
Full Liquid	Clear liquids plus milk products, eggs	Transition from clear to regular diet
Soft	Soft consistency and mild spice	Difficulty swallowing
Mechanical Soft	Regular diet but chopped or ground	Difficulty chewing
Bland	No spicy food	Ulcers or colitis
Low Residue	No bulky food, apples, or nuts	Rectal disease
High Calorie	High protein, vitamin, and fat	Malnourished

Continued.

Types of Diets—cont'd

Type	Description	Client Complaint
Low Calorie	Decreased fat, no whole milk, cream, eggs, complex carbohydrates	Obese
Diabetic	Balance of protein, carbohydrates, fat	Insulin-food imbalance
High Protein	Meat, fish, milk, cheese, poultry, eggs	Tissue repair, underweight
Low Fat	Little butter, cream, whole milk, or eggs	Gallbladder, liver, or heart disease
Low Cholesterol	Little meat or cheese	Need to decrease fat intake
Low Sodium	No salt added during cooking	Heart or renal disease
Salt Free	No salt	Heart or renal disease
Tube Feeding	Formulas or liquid food	Oral surgery, oral or esophageal cancers, inability to eat or swallow

Types of Nutrients		
Type	**Function**	**Food Sources**
Carbohydrate	Energy, body temperature	Simple: sugars, fruits, and nuts Complex: grains, potatoes, milk
Protein	Tissue growth, tissue repair	Meat, fish, eggs, milk poultry, beans, peas, nuts
Fat	Energy and repair, carries vitamins A and D	Animal fat, meat, nuts milk, fish, poultry
Water	Carries nutrients, regulates body processes, lubricates joints	Liquids, most fruits and vegetables

Minerals		
Type	**Function**	**Food Sources**
Calcium	Renews bones and teeth, regulates heart and nerves	Milk, green vegetables, cheese, salmon, legumes
Phosphorus	Renews bones and teeth, maintains nerve function	Cheese, oats, meat, milk, fish, poultry, nuts
Iron	Renews hemoglobin	Meat, eggs, liver, flour, yellow or green vegetables
Iodine	Regulates thyroid	Table salt, seafood
Magnesium	Component of enzymes	Grains, green vegetables
Sodium	Maintains water balance, nerve function	Salt, cured meats
Potassium	Maintains nerve function	Meat, milk, vegetables
Chloride	Formation of gastric juices	Salt
Zinc	Component of enzymes	Meat, seafood

	Vitamins	
Type	**Function**	**Food Sources**
A (Retinol)	Helps eyes, skin, hair, fights infection	Yellow fruits and vegetables, liver, kidneys, fish
B$_1$ (Thiamine)	Maintains nerves, aids carbohydrate function	Bread, cereal, beans, peas, pork, liver, eggs, milk
B$_2$ (Riboflavin)	Maintains skin, mouth, nerve functions	Milk, cheese, eggs, cereal, dark green vegetables
B$_3$ (Niacin)	Oxidation of proteins and carbohydrates	Meat, fish, poultry, eggs, nuts, bread, cereal
B$_{12}$	Aids muscles, nerves, heart, metabolism	Organ meats, milk
C (Ascorbic Acid)	Maintains integrity of cells, repairs tissue	Citrus fruits, tomatoes, green vegetables, potatoes
D	Enables body to use calcium and phosphorus	Milk, margarine, fish, liver, eggs
E	Antioxidant	Peanuts, vegetable oils
K	Aids in blood clotting	Green leafy vegetables

ALTERED BOWEL ELIMINATION PATTERNS

Constipation

Presence of large quantity of dry, hard feces that is difficult to expel. Frequency of bowel movements is not a factor.

Causes. Reabsorption of too much water in the lower bowel as a result of medications such as narcotics, ignoring the urge to defecate, immobility, chronic laxative abuse, low fluid intake, low fiber intake, aging, postoperative conditions or pregnancy.

Remedies. Increase fluids, fiber cereals, fruits and vegetables, and exercise and avoid cheese.

Impaction

Hard, dry stool embedded in rectal folds. May have liquid stool passing around impaction.

Causes. Poor bowel habits, immobility, inadequate food or fluids, or barium in rectum.

Remedies. Digitally remove impaction, increase fluids and fiber, increase exercise, and institute bowel program.

Diarrhea

Expulsion of fecal matter that contains too much water.

Causes. Infection, anxiety, stress, medications, too many laxatives at one time, or food or drug allergies or reactions.

Remedies. Add bulk or fiber to diet, maintain fluids and electrolytes, eat smaller amounts of food at one time, add cheese or bananas to diet, and rest after eating.

Incontinence

Inability to hold feces in rectum because of impairment of sphincter control.

Causes. Surgery, cancer, radiation treatment of rectum, paralysis, or aging.

Remedies. Bowel training, regular meal times, regular elimination patterns.

Abdominal Distention

Tympanites, or enlargement of the abdomen with gas or air as a result of excessive swallowing of air, eating gas-producing foods, or an inability to expel gas.

Causes. Constipation, fecal impaction, or postoperative conditions.

Remedy. Rectal tube can be used to expel air; increase ambulation, and change position in bed.

Obstruction

Occurs when the lumen of the bowel narrows or closes completely.

Causes. External compression can be caused by tumor, internal narrowing can be caused by impacted feces.

Remedies. Remove impaction or tumor.

Ileus

Occurs when the bowel has decreased motility.

Causes. Surgery, long-term narcotic use, or complete obstruction.

Remedies. Medical intervention of physical obstructions. Specific action will depend on the cause of the ileus.

Fecal Characteristics

Characteristic	Normal	Abnormal	Assess For
Color	Brown	Clay/white	Bile obstruction
		Black/tarry	Upper GI bleeding, iron
		Red	Lower GI bleeding, beets
		Pale	Malabsorption of fat
		Green	Infection
Consistency	Moist	Hard	Constipation, dehydration
	Formed	Loose	Diet, diarrhea, medications
		Watery	Infection
		Liquid	Impaction
Odor	Aromatic	Pungent	Infection, blood
Frequency	1-2 times per day	5 times per day	Infection, diet
	Once every 3 days	Once every 6 days	Constipation, activity, medications
Shape	Cylindrical	Narrow, "ribbon-like"	Obstruction

TYPES OF CATHARTICS

Bulk-forming increases fluids and bulk in the intestines, which stimulates peristalsis. An increase of fluid is needed.

   Example Metamucil

Emollient softens and delays drying of stool.

   Example liquid petrolatum

Irritant stimulates peristalsis by irritating bowel mucosa and decreasing water absorption.

   Example castor oil

Moistening (stool softeners) increases water in the bowel.

   Example Colace

Saline when salt is in the bowel the water will remain in the bowel as well. (Avoid use with clients with impaired renal function.)

   Example Milk of Magnesia (MOM), Epsom salts

Suppository stimulates bowel and softens stool.

ANTIDIARRHEAL MEDICATIONS

Demulcent coats and protects bowel

Absorbent absorbs gas

Astringents shrinks inflamed tissues

TYPES OF ENEMAS

Cleansing stimulates peristalsis, irritates bowel by distention. (Use 1 liter of fluid; have client hold it as long as possible.)

Carminative used to expel flatus.

Retention oil given to soften stool (hold for 1 hour).

Colonic irrigation used to expel flatus.

Hypertonic phosphates irritate bowel and draw fluid into bowel by osmosis (90 to 120 ml—hold 10 to 15 minutes).

Hypotonic tap water (1 liter—hold 15 minutes). Avoid with cardiac patients.

Soapsuds Irritates and distends bowel (5 ml of soap to 1 liter of water—hold 15 minutes). Use only castile soaps.

Saline draws fluid into the bowel (9 ml of sodium to 1 liter of water—hold 15 minutes).

Medicated contains a therapeutic agent (for example, Kayexalate to treat high potassium levels).

COMMON TYPES OF OSTOMIES*

Ileostomy

Effluent. A continuous discharge that is soft and wet. The output is somewhat odorous and contains intestinal enzymes that are irritating to peristomal skin.

Skin Barrier Option. Highly desirable for peristomal skin protection.

Pouch Option. Pouch necessary at all times.

Type of Pouch. Drainable or Closed-End for specific needs.

Need for Irrigation. None.

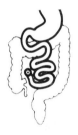

Transverse Colostomy

Effluent. Usually semiliquid or very soft. Occasionally, transverse colostomy discharge is firm. Output is usually malodorous and can irritate peristomal skin. Double-barreled colostomies have two openings. Loop colostomies have one opening, but two tracks—the active (proximal), which discharges fecal matter, and the inactive (distal), with a mucous discharge.

Skin Barrier Option. Highly desirable for peristomal skin protection.

Pouch Option. Pouch necessary at all times.

Type of Pouch. Drainable or Closed-End for specific needs.

Need for Irrigation. None.

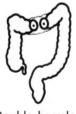 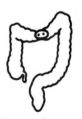

Double-barreled colostomy   Loop colostomy

Descending Colostomy/Sigmoid Colostomy

Effluent. Semisolid from descending colostomy. Firm from sigmoid colostomy. Upon discharge there is an odor. Discharge irritating if left in contact with skin around stoma. Frequency of output is unpredictable and varies with each person.

Skin Barrier Option. May be used for peristomal skin protection if pouch is worn.

Pouch Option. Pouch should be worn if person does not irrigate.

Type of Pouch. Drainable, Closed-End, or Stoma Cap.

Need for Irrigation. Yes, as instructed by ET nurse or physician.

Descending colostomy   Sigmoid colostomy

Urinary Diversion (Ileal Loop, Ileal, or Colonic Conduit)

Effluent. Urine only. Output is constant. Mucus is expelled with urine. Mild odor unless there is a urinary tract infection. Urine irritating when in contact with skin. Segment of ileum or colon is used to construct stoma.

Skin Barrier Option. Highly desirable for peristomal skin protection.

Pouch Option. Pouch necessary at all times.

Type of Pouch. Drainable pouch with spout.

Need for Irrigation. None.

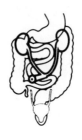

Continent Ileostomy

Effluent. Fluid bowel secretions are collected in a reservoir surgically constructed out of the lower part of the small intestine. Gas and feces are emptied via a surgically created leak-free nipple valve through which a catheter is inserted into the reservoir. For maximum efficiency and comfort, reservoir is usually emptied 4 to 5 times daily. Daily schedule for catheterization should be recommended by ET nurse or physician.

Skin Barrier Option. None. An absorbent pad will provide peristomal skin protection.

Pouch Option. None—but a catheter should be available at all times.

Type of Pouch. None. A drainable pouch can be applied if there is leakage of stool between intubations.

Need for Irrigation. Occasionally, to liquify thick fecal matter, the pouch can be irrigated with 1 to 1½ oz of saline or water. Specific care should be clarified by ET nurse or physician.

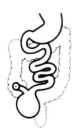

Continent Urostomy

Effluent. Urine is maintained in a surgically constructed ileal pouch until emptied by means of a catheter inserted into the stoma. Utilizes two nipple valves—one to prevent the reflux of urine from backing up into the kidneys, the other to keep urine in the pouch until eliminated. Pouch is drained approximately 4 times daily. Daily schedule for pouch catheterization should be recommended by ET nurse or physician.

Skin Barrier Option. None. An absorbent pad will provide peristomal skin protection.

Pouch Option. None—but a catheter should be available at all times.

Type of Pouch. None. A urostomy pouch can be applied if there is leakage of urine between intubations.

Need for Irrigation. Irrigate daily with 1 to 1½ oz of saline solution and repeat several times as needed until the returns are clear. Specific care should be clarified by ET nurse or physician.

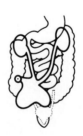

CHAPTER 14

Urinary System

Organs of the Urinary System
Altered Urinary Patterns
Urine Characteristics
Timed Urine Tests

For a more in-depth study of the urinary system consult the following publications:

AJN/Mosby: *Nursing boards review for the NCLEX-RN examination,* ed 9, St Louis, 1993, Mosby.

Anderson KN, Anderson LE: *Mosby's pocket dictionary of medicine, nursing, and allied health,* St Louis, 1994, Mosby.

Austrin MG, Austrin HR: *Learning medical terminology,* ed 7, St Louis, 1991, Mosby.

Phipps WJ, Long BC, Woods NF: *Medical-surgical nursing: concepts and clinical practice,* ed 4, St Louis, 1991, Mosby.

Potter PA, Perry AG: *Fundamentals of nursing: concepts, process, and practice,* ed 3, St Louis, 1993, Mosby.

ORGANS OF THE URINARY SYSTEM

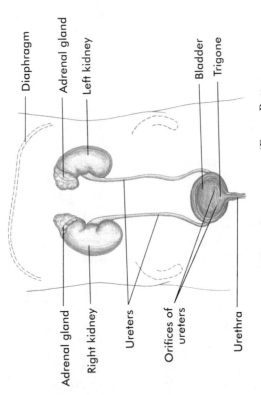

Figure 14-1 Organs of the urinary system. (From Potter PA, Perry AG: *Fundamentals of nursing*, ed 3, St Louis, 1993, Mosby.)

Altered Urinary Patterns		
Pattern	**Description**	**Assess For**
Anuria	No urination	Renal failure, dehydration, obstruction
Dysuria	Painful urination	Infection, injury, frequency, blood
Frequency	Voiding small amounts	Infection, injury, pregnancy, stress, intake
Incontinence	Difficulty with control	Infection, injury, distended bladder
Nocturia	Urinating at night	Infection, injury, pregnancy, stress, intake
Oliguria	Little urination	Infection, injury, BUN, dehydration, kidney disease
Polyuria	Increased urination	Infection, injury, alcohol, diabetes, caffeine, diuretics, increased thirst, dehydration
Retention	Holding on to urine	Infection, injury, pain, distended bladder, medications, restlessness, surgical complications
Residual	Urine remaining in bladder after voiding	Infection, distention, pain, injury
Urgency	Urgent and immediate need to void	Infection, injury, pregnancy, stress, intake

Urine Characteristics

Characteristics	Normal	Abnormal	Assess For
Amount in 24 hrs	1200 ml	<1200 ml	Renal failure
	1500 ml	>1500 ml	Fluid intake
Color	Straw	Amber	Dehydration, fluid intake
		Light straw	Overhydration
		Orange	Medications
		Red	Blood, injury, medications
Consistency	Clear	Cloudy	Infection
		Thick	Infection
Odor	Faint	Offensive	Infection, medications
Sterile	Yes	Organisms	Infection, poor hygiene
pH	4.5	<4.5	Infection
	8.0	>8.0	Diabetes, starvation, dehydration
Specific gravity	1.010	<1.010	Diabetes insipidus, kidney failure
	1.025	>1.025	Diabetes, underhydration
Glucose	None	Present	Diabetes
Ketones	None	Present	Diabetes, starvation, vomiting
Blood	None	Present	Tumors, injury, kidney disease

TIMED URINE TESTS

Quantitative albumin (24 hours) determines albumin lost in urine as a result of kidney disease, hypertension, or heart failure.

Amino acid (24 hours) determines presence of congenital kidney disease.

Amylase (2, 12, and 24 hours) determines presence of disease of the pancreas.

Chloride (24 hours) determines loss of chloride in cardiac patients on low-salt or no-salt diets.

Concentration and dilution determines presence of diseases of the kidney tubules.

Creatinine clearance (12 and 24 hours) determines the ability of the kidney to clear creatinine.

Estriol (24 hours) measures this hormone in women with high-risk pregnancies caused by diabetes.

Glucose tolerance (12 and 24 hours) determines malfunctions of the liver and pancreas.

17-Hydroxycorticosteroid (24 hours) determines functioning ability of the adrenal cortex.

Urinalysis (random times) determines levels of bacteria, WBCs, RBCs, pH, specific gravity, protein, and bilirubin.

Urine culture (random times) determines amount and type of bacteria in the urine.

Urine sensitivity (random times) determines which antibiotics the microoranisms will be sensitive or resistant to.

Urobilinogen (random times) determines presence of obstruction of the biliary tract.

CHAPTER 15

Reproductive System

Male Structures
Female Structures
Assessing Sexual History
Medications That Affect Sexual Performance
Common Male Reproductive Disorders
Common Female Reproductive Disorders
Sexually Transmitted Diseases

For a more in-depth study of the reproductive system consult the following publications:

AJN/Mosby: *Nursing boards review for the NCLEX-RN examination,* ed 9, St Louis, 1993, Mosby.

Anderson KN, Anderson LE: *Mosby's pocket dictionary of medicine, nursing, and allied health,* St Louis, 1994, Mosby.

Austrin MG, Austrin HR: *Learning medical terminology,* ed 7, St Louis, 1991, Mosby.

Phipps WJ, Long BC, Woods NF: *Medical-surgical nursing: concepts and clinical practice,* ed 4, St Louis, 1991, Mosby.

Potter PA, Perry AG: *Fundamentals of nursing: concepts, process, and practice,* ed 3, St Louis, 1993, Mosby.

MALE STRUCTURES

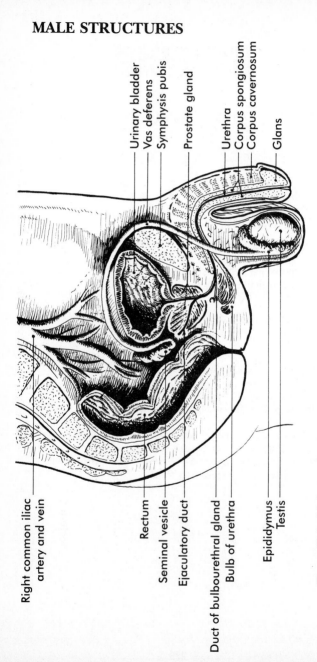

Figure 15-1 Male genitourinary system. (From Austrin MG, Austrin HR: *Learning medical terminology*, ed 7, St Louis, 1991, Mosby.)

Urinary bladder
Vas deferens
Symphysis pubis
Prostate gland
Urethra
Corpus spongiosum
Corpus cavernosum
Glans

Right common iliac artery and vein

Rectum
Seminal vesicle
Ejaculatory duct
Duct of bulbourethral gland
Bulb of urethra
Epididymus
Testis

FEMALE STRUCTURES

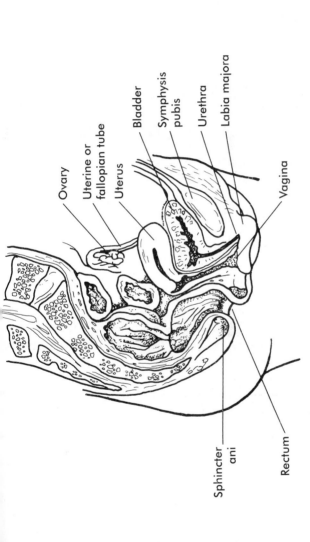

Figure 15-2 Female reproductive system. (From Austrin MG, Austrin HR: *Learning medical terminology*, ed 7, St Louis, 1991, Mosby.)

ASSESSING SEXUAL HISTORY

Include the following:

Male

Practice of testicular examinations.
Last prostate exam and results.
Knowledge of deficit.
Concerns or difficulty with sexual activities.
Body image concerns.
Concerns regarding the effect of treatment on future sexual activities.
Attitudes regarding sex.

Female

Last menstrual cycle.
Onset of menopause.
Knowledge deficit.
Number of children, pregnancies, and miscarriages.
Body image concerns.
Practice of breast self-examination.
Last mammogram and results.
Last Pap smear and pelvic examination and results.
Any concerns or difficulty with sexual activities.
Concerns regarding the effect of treatment on future sexual activities.
Attitudes regarding sex.

MEDICATIONS THAT AFFECT SEXUAL PERFORMANCE

Antidepressants blurred vision, confusion, and loss of desire

Antihypertensives loss of desire, weakness

Antiemetics impotence, restlessness, and insomnia

Cimetidine impotence, dizziness, headaches, and nausea

Diuretics dizziness, headaches, and weakness

Oral contraceptives allow for sexual activity without concern about conception

Ranitidine impotence, dizziness, headaches, and nausea

Steroids mood changes, menstrual changes, headaches, and weakness

Tranquilizers drowsiness, confusion, and decreased sexual desire

Common Male Reproductive Disorders

Disorder	Description	Assess For
Hydrocele	Collection of fluid in testes	Pain, swelling
Spermatocele	Cystic mass of the epididymis	Pain, swelling
Varicocele	Dilation of spermatic vein	Pain, swelling
Torsion of spermatic cord	Kinking of cord	Sexual dysfunction
Cancer	Testicular cancer	Enlarged testes, lump
	Penile cancer	Growths, fatigue, weight loss, dysfunction
	Prostate cancer	Urinary dysfunction
Urethritis	Inflammation of urethra	Urgency, frequency, burning with urination
Prostatitis	Inflammation of prostate	Pain, fever, dysuria, urethral drainage
Epididymitis	Inflammation of epididymis	Scrotal pain, edema
Benign prostatic hypertrophy	Enlarged prostate	Dysuria, pain

Common Female Reproductive Disorders

Disorder	Description	Assess For
Uterine prolapse	Displacement of uterus	Dysmenorrhea, backache, pelvic pain
Cystocele	Bladder herniation into vagina	Backache, stress incontinence
Rectocele	Rectum herniation into vagina	Constipation, hemorrhoids
Ovarian cyst	Enlarged ovaries	Menstrual changes, abdominal swelling
Endometriosis	Seeding of endometrial cells into pelvis	Pain, infertility, menstrual changes
Cervical polyps	Benign tumor	Bleeding between periods and with intercourse, increased cervical mucosa
Cancer	Cervical cancer	Spotting, pain
	Uterine cancer	Pain, abdominal fullness, postmenopausal bleeding
	Ovarian cancer	Ascites, fatigue, weight loss, abdominal fullness

	Sexually Transmitted Diseases*		
Organism	Diseases	Symptoms	Treatment
Bacteria	Gonorrhea, chancroid, granuloma	Purulent discharge	Penicillin
Spirochete	Syphilis	Stage 1: chancre Stage 2: body rash Stage 3: tumors, nerve damage, cardiac damage	Penicillin

*Sexually transmitted diseases are any disorders that can be transmitted from one person to another during sexual contact.

Sexually Transmitted Diseases—cont'd

Organism	Diseases	Symptoms	Treatment
Chlamydia	Nongonococcal urethritis, cervicitis, epididymitis, pelvic inflammatory disease	Purulent drainage, fever, chills, pain, and vomiting	Antibiotics
Virus	Herpes, cytomegalovirus (HPV)	Vesicles	Acyclovir
	AIDS	Pulmonary infections	Antibiotics, supportive care
Protozoa	Trichomoniasis	Itching, greenish discharge	Vinegar
Yeast	Candidiasis	Itching, white, cheesy discharge	Nystatin, miconazole

CHAPTER 16

Tests and Procedures

For a more in-depth study of tests and procedures consult the following publications:

AJN/Mosby: *Nursing boards review for the NCLEX-RN examination,* ed 9, St Louis, 1993, Mosby.

Anderson KN, Anderson LE: *Mosby's pocket dictionary of medicine, nursing, and allied health,* St Louis, 1994, Mosby.

Austrin MG, Austrin HR: *Learning medical terminology,* ed 7, St Louis, 1991, Mosby.

Myers JL: *Quick medication administration reference,* St Louis, 1992, Mosby.

Pagana KD, Pagana TJ: *Mosby's diagnostic and laboratory test reference,* St Louis, 1992, Mosby.

Phipps WJ, Long BC, Woods NF: *Medical-surgical nursing: concepts and clinical practice,* ed 4, St Louis, 1991, Mosby.

Potter PA, Perry AG: *Fundamentals of nursing: concepts, process, and practice,* ed 3, St Louis, 1993, Mosby.

LABORATORY VALUES*

Complete Blood Count

Red blood cells (RBC)	$4.25\text{-}6.1 \times 10$/ml (males)
	$3.6\text{-}5.4 \times 10$/ml (females)
White blood cells (WBC)	$5000\text{-}10,000$/mm^3
Hemoglobin (Hgb)	13-18 g/dl (males)
	12-16 g/dl (females)
Hematocrit (Hct)	45%-54% (males)
	37%-47% (females)

Coagulation

Platelet	150,000-350,000/ml
Prothrombin time (PT)	10-14 sec
Partial thromboplastin time (PTT)	30-45 sec
Thrombin time (TT)	Control ± 5 sec
Fibrinogen split products (FSP)	Negative reaction at >1:4 dilution
Iron/ferritin (Fe) (deficiency)	0-20 ng/ml
Reticulocyte count	0.5%-1.5% of red cells

*Averages may vary per facility.

Blood Chemistry

Sodium (Na)	135-145 mEq/L
Potassium (K)	3.5-4.5 mEq/L
Chloride (Cl)	98-106 mEq/L
Carbon dioxide (CO_2)	24-32 mEq/L
Blood urea nitrogen (BUN)	7-25 mg/dl
Creatinine (Cr)	0.7-1.3 mg/dl (males)
	0.6-1.2 mg/dl (females)
Glucose	70-110 mg/dl
Calcium (Ca)	8.5-10.5 mg/dl
Magnesium (Mg)	1.3-2.1 mg/dl
Phosphorus	3.0-4.5 mg/dl
Osmolality	275-295 mOsm/kg
Bilirubin	
Direct	0-0.2 mg/dl
Total	0.2-1.0 mg/dl
Indirect is total minus direct	
Amylase	50-150 U/L
Lipase	0-110 U/L
Anion gap	8-16 mEq/L

Urine Electrolytes

Sodium (Na)	40-220 mEq/L
Potassium (K)	25-125 mEq/L
Chloride (Cl)	110-250 mEq/L

ARTERIAL BLOOD GASES

Acid-base balance (pH) measures hydrogen concentration (7.35-7.45).

Oxygenation (Pao$_2$) measures partial pressure of dissolved oxygen in the blood (80-100 mm Hg).

Saturation (So$_2$) measures percentage of O$_2$ to hemoglobin (95%-98%).

Ventilation (Paco$_2$) measures partial pressure of CO$_2$ (38-45 mm Hg).

Nursing Interventions
Preparation

Cleanse the area over the artery with an iodine cleaner. Collect an ABG syringe, needle, and heparin.

Collection

An ABG test must be done by a physician, specially trained nurse, or laboratory technician. Keep the client calm.

PostABG

The sample will need to go the laboratory immediately. Some facilities may require an advance call to the laboratory before an ABG test specimen can be sent.

Acid-Base Imbalances

Clinical Manifestations

Acidosis	Alkalosis

Respiratory Manifestations
Causes

Carbonic excess, pneumonia, hypoventilation, obesity

Carbonic deficit, anxiety, fear, hyperventilation, anemia, asthma

Signs and Symptoms

Confusion/CNS depression

Unconsciousness (late sign)

Laboratory Values

pH 7.25 (low)
$Paco_2$ 60 mm Hg (high)
Bicarbonate normal
Pao_2 60 mm Hg (acute)
Pao_2 80 mm Hg (chronic)

pH 7.52 (high)
$Paco_2$ 31 mm Hg (low)
Bicarbonate normal
Pao_2 90 mm Hg (high)

Continued.

Acid-Base Imbalances—cont'd	
Clinical Manifestations	
Acidosis	**Alkalosis**

Metabolic Manifestations
Causes

Bicarbonate deficit, ketoacidosis, starvation, shock, diarrhea, renal failure	Bicarbonate excess, Cushing's syndrome, hypokalemia, hypercalcemia, excessive vomiting, diuretics

Signs and Symptoms

Weakness, disorientation, coma	Respiratory depression, tetany, mental dullness

Laboratory Values

pH <7.35	pH >7.45
Urine pH <6	Urine pH >7
$Paco_2$ normal	$Paco_2$ normal
K+ >5	K+ <3.5
Bicarbonate <21 mEq/L	Bicarbonate >28 mEq/L

ELECTROLYTE IMBALANCES

Clinical Manifestations

Hyponatremia (<135 mEq/L)

Signs and Symptoms. Fatigue, abdominal cramps, diarrhea, weakness, hypotension, cool, clammy skin.
Causes. Overhydration, kidney disease, diarrhea.

Hypernatremia (>145 mEq/L)

Signs and Symptoms. Thirst, dry, sticky mucous membranes, dry tongue and skin, flushed skin, increased body temperature.
Causes. Dehydration, starvation, (SIADH)

Hypokalemia (<3.5 mEq/L)

Signs and Symptoms. Weakness, fatigue, anorexia, abdominal distention, dysrhythmias, decreased bowel sounds.
Causes. Diarrhea, diuretics, alkalosis, polyuria.

Hyperkalemia (>5 mEq/L)

Signs and Symptoms. Anxiety, dysrhythmias, increased bowel sounds.
Causes. Burns, renal failure, dehydration, acidosis.

Hypocalcemia (<8.3 mEq/L)

Signs and Symptoms. Abdominal cramps, tingling, muscle spasms, convulsions. Assess magnesium level.
Causes. Parathyroid dysfunction, vitamin D deficiency, pancreatitis.

Hypercalcemia (>10 mEq/L)

Signs and Symptoms. Deep bone pain, nausea, vomiting, constipation. Assess magnesium level.
Causes. Parathyroid tumor, bone cancer/metastasis, osteoporosis.

Hypomagnesemia (<1.3 mEq/L)

Signs and Symptoms. Tremors, muscle cramps, tachycardia, hypertension, confusion. Assess calcium level.
Causes. Parathyroid dysfunction, cancer, chemotherapy, polyuria.

Hypermagnesemia (>2.5 mEq/L)

Signs and Symptoms. Lethargy, respiratory difficulty, coma. Assess calcium level.
Causes. Parathyroid dysfunction, renal failure.

FLUID VOLUME IMBALANCES

Fluid Volume Deficit (Hypovolemia)

Signs and Symptoms. Hypotension, weight loss, decreased tearing or saliva, dry skin or mouth, oliguria, increased pulse or respirations, increased specific gravity of urine, increased serum sodium levels.

Causes. Dehydration, insufficient fluid intake, diuretics, sweating or polyuria, excessive tube feedings leading to diarrhea.

Fluid Volume Excess (Hypervolemia)

Signs and Symptoms. Edema, puffy face or eyelids, ascites, rales or wheezes in lungs, bounding pulse, hypertension, sudden weight gain, decreased serum sodium levels.

Causes. Overhydration, renal failure, congestive heart failure.

Common Fluid Volumes*

Small glass of water: 200 ml	Juice: 120 ml
Small bowl of soup: 180 ml	Teapot: 240 ml
Water pitcher: 1 L	Gelatin: 120 ml
Ice cream: 120 ml	Medium cup: 30 ml

Common IV Solutions

Normal saline—0.9% saline (NS)
5% Dextrose in water (D_5W)
5% Dextrose in 0.9% saline (D_5 NS)
5% Dextrose in 0.45% saline (D_5 ½ NS)
Lactated Ringer's (NaCl, K+, Ca++, lactic acid)

*Volumes may vary per institution.

DIAGNOSTIC TESTS

Angiography records cardiac pressures, function, and output (client may need special postprocedure vital signs taken).

Arterial blood gases measurements of arterial blood pH, Po_2, $Paco_2$, and bicarbonate (blood sample needs to be kept on ice).

Arteriography x-ray examination with injections of dye used to locate occlusions (client may need special postprocedure vital signs taken).

Arthrography x-ray examination of the bones.

Barium study x-ray examination to locate polyps, tumors, or other colon problems (barium needs to be removed after procedure).

Barium swallow detects esophageal narrowing, varices, strictures, or tumors (barium needs to be removed after procedure).

Biopsy removal of specific tissue (assess client for pain after procedure).

Blood tests (see section on laboratory values for normal values.)

Bone marrow biopsy examination of a piece of tissue from bone marrow (assess client for pain after procedure).

Bone scan radioisotope used to locate tumors or other bone disorders (client must be able to lie flat).

Brain scan radioisotope used to locate tumors, strokes, or seizure disorders (client must lie flat).

Bronchoscopy inspection of the larynx, trachea, and bronchi with flexible scope (client may need sedation).

Cardiac catheterization uses dye to visualize heart's arteries (client may need special postprocedure vital signs taken).

Chest x-ray used to look for pneumonia, cancer, and other diseases of the lung.

Cholangiography x-ray examination of the biliary ducts.

Cholecystography x-ray examination of the gallbladder.

Colonoscopy uses flexible scope to view colon (client may need to be sedated).

Colposcopy examination of the cervix and vagina.

Computerized tomography (CT scan) three dimensional x-ray (client must be able to lie flat).

Culdoscopy flexible tube used to view pelvic organs.

Culture and sensitivity determines source and type of bacteria.

Cystoscopy direct visualization of bladder with cystoscope.

Dilatation and curettage dilatation of the cervix followed by endometrial cleansing (done in surgery).

Doppler ultrasound used to show venous or arterial patency.

Echocardiography ultrasound that records structure and functions of the heart.

Electrocardiography records electrical impulses generated by the heart.

Electroencephalography records electrical activity of the brain (client should be resting).

Electromyography records electrical activity of the muscles.

Endoscopy inspection of upper GI with flexible scope (client may need to be sedated).

Endoscopic retrograde cholangiopancreatography (ERCP) x-ray examination of the gallbladder and pancreas.

Exercise stress test recording of the heart rate, activity, and blood pressure while the body is at work.

Fluoroscopy x-ray examination with picture displayed on television monitor.

GI series x-ray examination using barium to locate ulcers (barium must be removed after procedure).

Hemoccult detects blood in stool, emesis, and elsewhere.

Holter monitor checks and records irregular heart rates and rhythms (generally over a 24 hour period).

Intravenous pyelography (IVP) x-ray examination of the kidneys after dye injection.

KUB x-ray examination of the kidneys, ureter, and bladder.

Laparoscopy abdominal examination with a flexible scope.

Lumbar puncture sampling of spinal fluid; often called a spinal tap (can be done bedside).

Magnetic resonance imaging (MRI) three-dimensional x-ray similar to CT scan.

Mammography x-ray examination of the breast.

Myelography injection of dye into subarachnoid space in order to view brain and spinal cord.

Pap smear detects cervical cancer.

Proctoscopy inspection of lower colon with flexible scope (client may need to be sedated).

Pulmonary function test (PFT) measures lung capacity and volume to detect problems.

Pyelography x-ray examination of kidneys.

Sigmoidoscopy inspection of lower colon with flexible scope (client may need to be sedated).

Small bowel follow-through (SBFT) done in addition to a GI series.

Spinal tap see Lumbar puncture

Thallium radionuclear dye used to assess heart functions.

Tuberculin skin test test for tuberculosis using tuberculin purified protein derivative (PPD).

Ultrasound reflection of sound waves.

Urine tests see Chapter 14.

Venography x-ray examination used to locate a thrombus in a vein.

CHAPTER 17

Surgical Nursing Care

For a more in-depth study of surgical nursing care consult the following publications:

Austrin MG, Austrin HR: *Learning medical terminology,* ed 7, St Louis, 1991, Mosby.

Phipps WJ, Long BC, Woods NF: *Medical-surgical nursing: concepts and clinical practice,* ed 4, St Louis, 1991, Mosby.

Potter PA, Perry AG: *Fundamentals of nursing: concepts, process, and practice,* ed 3, St Louis, 1993, Mosby.

NURSING CARE BEFORE SURGERY

Teaching

Include the following:

Smoking or drinking restrictions before surgery.

Dietary or fluid restrictions before surgery.

Review of surgical procedure.

Postoperative deep breathing, positioning, and ROM exercises.

Postoperative pain and pain relief measures available.

Postoperative activity or dietary restrictions.

Postoperative dressing procedures.

Review of drains, nasogastric, catheter, and IVs that may be inserted during surgery.

History

Include the following:

Chief complaint or reason for surgery.

Prior surgeries and responses or impressions.

Drug allergies.

Physical limitations such as vision or hearing problems, limps, or paralysis.

History of smoking and drinking (last drink or food intake).

Medications and the last time taken.

Nonprescription or recreational drug use and when taken last.

History of strokes, heart attacks, seizures, diabetes, and thyroid or adrenal diseases.

Concerns, questions, or special requests.

Significant others and where they can be reached after surgery.

Checklist

Include the following:

Signed consent form in the front of the chart.

List of clothes and valuables and their placement in a safe place.

Record of vital signs and last time voided.

List of prostheses such as dentures and limbs (removed).

List of preoperative medications and when administered.

Review of preoperative laboratory values and tests.

Preoperative surgical scrubbing (Figures 17-1 and 17-2).

Review of Body Systems

Note any problems, including the following:

Cardiac dysrhythmia, edema, cyanosis, chest pain, hypertension, murmur, heart rate, blood pressure.

Respiratory cough, shortness of breath, dyspnea, wheezing, orthopnea orthostasis, diminished sounds, rate, depth.

Neurologic headaches, dizziness, ringing in ears, gait, reflexes, muscle strength, emotions.

Gastrointestinal nausea, vomiting, weight gain or loss, ulcers, Crohn's disease or ulcerative colitis, devices.

Genitourinary urgency, frequency, retention, urinary tract infections, need for Foley catheter or other devices.

Skin bruising, open sores, rashes, signs of infection, general condition.

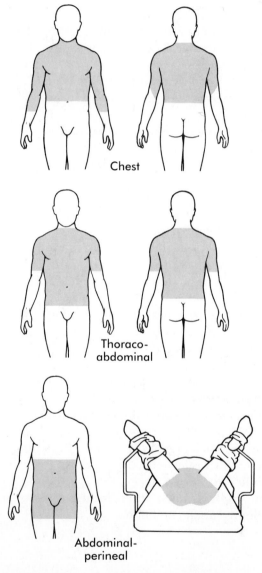

Figure 17-1 Surgical skin preparations.

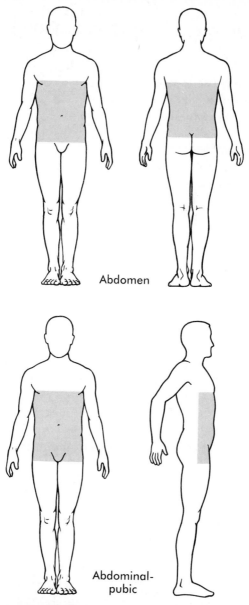

Abdomen

Abdominal-
pubic

Figure 17-2 Surgical skin preparations.

NURSING CARE AFTER SURGERY

Objectives
Provide a safe environment for the client.
Monitor the client's condition.
Recognize potential complications.

Information Needed*
Type of surgery and anesthetic.
Findings and results of the surgery.
Any complications during the surgery.
Transfusions given to the client.
Current respiratory condition of the client.
Current cardiac and circulatory condition of the client.
Types and number of incisions, drains, tubes, and IVs.
Current vital signs and when they need to be taken next.
Current laboratory values and when specimens need to be drawn next.
Dressing location, condition, and changes (the first change is generally done by the surgeon).
Neurologic status and need for future neurologic checks.
Time, frequency, and route of administration of pain medications.
Additional postoperative orders.
Notify any family or significant others waiting for the client.

*Can be found in the chart.

CARE OF BODY SYSTEMS AFTER SURGERY

Cardiac

Possibility of hemorrhage, shock, embolism, thrombosis.

Monitor blood pressure, heart rate, rhythm, quality.

Check for Homans' sign, leg tenderness, leg edema.

Check capillary refill, hemorrhage, shock, pedal pulses.

Pulmonary

Possibility of obstruction, atelectasis, pneumonia.

Turn client every 1 to 2 hours unless contraindicated.

Have client cough and deep breathe using pillows to splint incisions.

Assess lungs for rales, rhonchi, or wheezes. Check oxygen saturation.

Perform oral or deep suction as needed. Have client use incentive spirometer as needed.

Use humidification to ease breathing, and chest therapy if ordered.

Ensure adequate hydration to help thin secretions, and postural drainage to drain secretions.

Assess for adequate pain relief to help breathing.

Neurologic

Perform neurologic and reflex checks as needed.

Assess orientation, level of consciousness, and pain control as needed.

Assess for restlessness, fatigue, and anxiety.

Explain the need for the procedures to the client.

Genitourinary

Assess for adequate fluid intake and output and for bladder distention.

Assess the need for and care of Foley catheter or need for straight catheterization.

Gastrointestinal

Assess bowel sounds for possible ileus (indicated by no sounds).

Assess for nausea, vomiting, distended abdomen, gas pains.

Skin

Assess wound for drainage and signs of infection.
Assess for skin breakdown.

TYPES OF DRESSINGS

Name	Uses
Absorbent	Drains wound (increases evaporation)
Antiseptic	Prevents infection
Dry	With wound with little or no drainage
Hot/Moist	Promotes wound healing by second or third intention; increases blood supply to wound
Occlusive	Prevents invasion of bacteria
Protective	Protects wound from injury
Wet to Damp	Dressing removed before wound drys
Wet to Dry	With open wound that has necrotic tissue; wounds with greatest drainage
Wet to Wet	With wound that needs to be kept very moist

COMMON SURGICAL PROCEDURES*

Anastomosis a creation of a passage between two vessels.

Angiectomy/angioplasty removal/repair of a vessel.

Aortotomy incision into the aorta.

Arteriectomy/arterioplasty removal/repair of an artery.

Arthrectomy/arthroplasty removal/repair of a joint.

Atriotomy incision into an atrium of the heart.

Biopsy incision to remove a tissue sample.

Bronchotomy/bronchoplasty incision into/repair of a bronchus.

Cholecystectomy removal of the gallbladder.

Choledochectomy removal of a portion of the common bile duct.

Colectomy partial removal of the colon.

Coronary artery bypass graft (CABG) a large vein from the body is removed and sutured to either side of an obstructed coronary artery.

Craniectomy/cranioplasty removal/repair of a portion of the skull.

Cystectomy/cystoplasty removal/repair of the bladder.

Dermabrasion surgical removal of epidermis or a portion of the dermis.

Embolization a suturing or sealing of a vessel.

Esophagectomy/esophagoplasty removal/repair of the esophagus.

Fasciectomy/fascioplasty removal/repair of the fascia.

Gastrectomy/gastroplasty removal/repair of the stomach.

*Refer to sections on prefixes and suffixes to build surgical vocabulary.

Graft surgical replacement of tissue, skin, or muscle.

Hysterectomy removal of the uterus.

Laminectomy removal of the posterior arch of a vertebra.

Laryngectomy/laryngoplasty removal/repair of the larynx.

Lymphangiectomy/lymphangioplasty removal/repair of a lymph vessel.

Mastectomy/mastopexy removal/reduction of a breast.

Myectomy/myoplasty removal/repair of a muscle.

Nephrectomy removal of a kidney.

Oophorectomy/oophoroplasty removal/repair of an ovary.

Orchiectomy/orchioplasty removal/repair of a testicle.

Osteoclasis reconstruction of a fractured bone.

Percutaneous transluminal coronary angioplasty (PTCA) a balloon procedure used to push an obstruction against a vessel wall to allow blood to flow through.

Pericardiectomy removal of the pericardium.

Phlebectomy/phleboplasty removal/repair of a vein.

Pneumonectomy removal of a lung.

Radical mastectomy removal of a breast, pectorals, lymph nodes, and skin.

Rhinoplasty plastic repair of the nose.

Splenotomy/splenorrhapy incision into/repair of the spleen.

Thoracoplasty removal of a rib to allow collapse of the lungs.

Valvulotomy/valvuloplasty incision into/repair of a valve.

RED BLOOD CELL TRANSFUSIONS

Typing selecting the ABO blood type and Rh antigen factor of a person's blood (other antigens can also affect transfusion compatibility.

Cross matching mixing the recipient's serum with the donor's red blood cells in a saline solution; if no agglutination occurs, the blood may be safely given.

Blood Type	Can Generally Donate To	Can Generally Receive From
A−	A−, A+	A−, O−
B−	B−, B+	B−, O−
AB−	AB−, AB+	AB−, A−, B−, O−
A+	A+	A+, A−, O+, O−
B+	B+	B+, B−, O+, O−
AB+	AB+	All Blood Types
O−	All Blood Types	O−
O+	O+, A+, B+, AB+	O+, O−

Before Administering Blood to a Client

Check facility's policy on infusing blood products.

Check the client's ID band for proper identification.

Check the client's blood type and Rh antigen.

Get the blood from blood bank only when ready to infuse.

Compare the client's blood type to the type of blood to be infused.

Two professionals must check and cosign blood.

Start infusion of blood with normal saline solution.

Administer blood at a slower rate for the first 15 minutes. Blood should be infused within 4 hours.

Use appropriate blood tubing and needles (may vary per facility).

Document action on appropriate flow sheets (may vary per facility).

Instruct client to report *any* discomfort (blood reactions).

Special vital signs are needed (may vary per facility).

Some facilities may medicate the client with acetaminophen or diphenhydramine (Benadryl) before infusion.

Blood Reactions

Possible reactions include difficulty breathing, wheezing, tachypnea, fever, tachycardia, change in blood pressure, chest pain, disorientation, rash, or hives. *If a reaction begins, stop the infusion.* Begin a normal saline flush to keep the IV line open and administer prescribed antihistamines. Notify a physician, recheck blood, retype, and crossmatch. *Do not* discard the blood—the laboratory may want to analyze it for the cause of the reaction. The physician may require a urine sample from the client.

CHAPTER 18

Client Safety

For a more in-depth study of client safety consult the following publications:

Phipps WJ, Long BC, Woods NF: *Medical-surgical nursing: concepts and clinical practice,* ed 4, St Louis, 1991, Mosby.

Potter PA, Perry AG: *Fundamentals of nursing: concepts, process, and practice,* ed 3, St Louis, 1993, Mosby.

ADMISSION SAFETY

The Client's Room

When a client is admitted to the hospital it is important that the client is aware of all equipment located in his or her room. This can prevent accidents and make the hospital stay safer. Point out the following items on admission:

Call light or bell, room lights, bathroom, bathroom lights, nurses' station, side rails, room number.

Make sure that the following equipment is working properly:

Call lights, side rails, bed controls, room lights, oxygen.

ONGOING SAFETY

To ensure ongoing safety take the following precautions:

Clear the client's room of excess debris.

No furniture should be blocking the doorway to the client's room.

Immediately clean up any water or other liquid spills on the floor.

Do not leave needles or other sharp items near the client.

Remove unmarked bottles and syringes from client's room.

Label all IV and central lines, nasogastric, gastrostomy, and jejunostomy tubes.

Check all electrical equipment for proper functioning and condition.

Double check all medications before giving them to the client, using the six client rights.

Double check the client ID bracelet before giving medications, performing any procedures, and transferring the client to another department for tests, another unit, surgery, or therapy appointments.

SPECIAL CLIENT SITUATIONS

Hospitalized clients with the following problems may require additional safety measures.

Alcohol Withdrawal

Signs and Symptoms. Confusion, sweating, pallor, palpitations, hypotension, seizures, coma. Protocols may vary by facility.

Withdrawal protocols may include seizure precautions, keeping the side rails up and padded, taking vital signs frequently (every 30 to 60 minutes or per hospital protocol), and close observation. Provide a safe environment. Perform neurologic, memory, or orientation checks. Document any withdrawal activity and actions taken.

Bleeding/Hemorrhage

Locate the source of the bleeding. Apply direct pressure with a clean drape. Call for assistance but stay with the client. Assess for early signs of shock such as changes in sensorium and later signs of shock such as hypotension, pale skin, and a rapid, weak pulse.

Prevention. Closely supervise confused or heavily medicated clients and clients just returning from surgery. Make sure surgical dressings are secure. Encourage clients to call for assistance if bleeding begins. Document any bleeding and actions taken.

Choking

Follow standard Heimlich maneuver guidelines.
Prevention. Closely supervise confused or heavily medicated clients. Make sure clients are sitting up or are placed in high Fowler's position when eating. Encourage the use of the call lights. Assess the client's ability to chew and swallow. Order a diet appropriate to the client's eating ability. Document any choking situations and actions taken.

Drug Reactions

Assess for difficulty breathing, wheezing, tearing, palpitations, skin rash, pruritus, nausea or vomiting, rhinitis, diarrhea, and a change in mood or mental status. *These are general drug reactions, not the side effects of specific drugs. Immediately report all drug reactions.*
Prevention. Closely supervise confused or heavily medicated clients, or those clients who are taking medications for the first time. Encourage the use of the call lights should any of the signs of a drug reaction occur. *Know your client's drug allergies.* Document all drug reactions and actions taken.

THE CONFUSED CLIENT

Assess for the source of the confusion. Possible sources include age, medications, disease, and infection. The confused client is at risk for falls.

Falls

Assess for the client's ability to ambulate, environment, mental status, and medications.

Prevention. Closely supervise confused or heavily medicated clients, encourage the use of the call lights or the use of night lights, raise side rails and encourage client to use grab bars or side rails, post a sign alerting others to the possibility of falls, lock wheelchairs, use gait belts, avoid water or other liquid spills, and use nonskid footwear.

Restraints

When to Use. To prevent injury to client or others, restrict movement, or immobilize a body part.

Types of Restraints. Jackets/vests, belts, mittens, wrist or ankle, crib net, and elbow.

Guidelines. Get physician's order and follow hospital protocol. Explain purpose of restraints to client, check circulation every 30 minutes, release temporarily (once an hour), and provide ROM. Document need for restraints, examination schedule, and use of ROM. Report problems and client's level of tolerance for restraints, and provide emotional support. *Never secure restraints to the side rails or the nonstationary portion of the main frame of the bed.*

Complications. Skin breakdown (pad bony areas); nerve damage (do not over-tighten restraints and release client from them often); circulatory impairment (check for problems often, and provide ROM exercises); and death (from inadequate or improper use of restraints).

EMERGENCIES

Fire

RACE—**R**escue clients, **A**lert others/pull **A**larm, **C**ontain fire, **E**xtinguish Fire. All extinguishers are labeled A, B, C, or D according to the types of fires they are meant to extinguish. Some extinguishers can be used for more than one type of fire and will be labeled with more than one letter. The types of fires the letters correspond to are:

A. Paper or wood   B. Liquid or gas
C. Electrical   D. Combustible metals

Any of the following emergencies may require CPR.

Heart Attack

Signs and Symptoms. Chest pain; shortness of breath; dyspnea; a squeezing, crushing, or heavy feeling in the chest; lightheadedness; pain in left arm or in the jaw; and nausea.

Intervention. Calm the client and turn on the call light. Begin oxygen at 2 liters if nearby. Remain calm and stay with the client until help arrives. Document symptoms and actions taken.

Pulmonary Embolism

Signs and Symptoms. Chest pain, shortness of breath, dyspnea, cyanosis, and possible death.
Causes. Immobility, deep vein thrombosis.
Intervention. Calm client and turn on the call light. Begin oxygen at 2 liters if nearby. Remain calm and stay with the client until help arrives. Document symptoms and actions taken.

Prevention. Elevate legs, use antiembolism stockings, dorsiflexion of foot, perform ROM exercises, check Homans' sign, perform coughing and deep breathing exercise, and administer low dosages of heparin as prescribed while client is hospitalized. Do not massage lower legs.

Cardiac Arrest

Remain calm and turn on the call light. Begin CPR (follow standard guidelines) until more experienced staff arrives and takes over. Clear furniture from the room and ask family to move to waiting area. (Some facilities will allow family to watch CPR activity.)

Seizures

Signs and Symptoms

Grand mal total body stiffness, staring, jerking muscles.

Petit mal daydreaming, staring.

Causes. Neurologic disease, cancer, head injury, fever or pregnancy-induced hypertension.

Interventions. Remain calm and turn on the call light. Ensure the client's safety, lower the bed, and raise side rails. Stay with the client, time the seizure, and make sure the client does not hit his or her head. Document seizure activity and actions taken.

Shock

Signs and Symptoms

Mild/early warm, flushed skin, changes in orientation, widening pulse pressure.

Moderate/mild cool, clammy, pale skin, hypotension, narrowing pulse pressure, sweating, pallor, rapid pulse, decrease in urinary output.

Severe/late all of the symptoms of moderate/mild shock plus irregular pulse, oliguria, shallow, rapid breathing, obtunded, or comatose.

Causes. Hemorrhage, infection, or hypovolemia.

Intervention. Monitor vital signs, assess orientation, and keep the client warm. Record all symptoms and vital signs.

REFERENCES

AJN/Mosby-*Nursing Boards Review for the NCLEX-RN examination,* ed 9, St Louis, 1993, Mosby.

Anderson KN, Anderson LE: *Mosby's pocket dictionary of medicine, nursing, and allied health,* St Louis, 1994, Mosby.

Austrin MG, Austrin HR: *Learning medical terminology,* ed 7, St Louis, 1991, Mosby.

Benenson AB, editor: *Control of communicable diseases in man,* Washington, D.C., 1990, American Public Health Association.

Conway-Rutkowski BL: *Carini and Owens' neurological and neurosurgical nursing,* ed 8, St Louis, 1982, Mosby.

Guzzetta CE, Dossey BM: *Cardiovascular nursing: holistic practice,* St Louis, 1992, Mosby.

Myers JL: *Quick medication administration reference,* St Louis, 1992, Mosby.

Pagana KD, Pagana TJ: *Mosby's diagnostic and laboratory test reference,* St Louis, 1992, Mosby.

Phipps WJ, Long BC, Woods NF: *Medical-surgical nursing: concepts and clinical practice,* ed 4, St Louis, 1991, Mosby.

Potter PA, Perry AG: *Fundamentals of nursing: concepts, process, and practice,* ed 3, St Louis, 1993, Mosby.

Skidmore-Roth L: *Mosby's nursing drug reference,* ed 6, St Louis, 1993, Mosby.

Sorrentino SA: *Mosby's textbook for nursing assistants,* St Louis, 1992, Mosby.

Williams SR: *Nutrition and diet therapy,* ed 7, St Louis, 1993, Mosby.

INDEX

NOTES

NOTES

NOTES

NOTES

NOTES

NOTES

NOTES

NOTES

NOTES